DETOXELICIOUS

EASY SOUL FOOD INSPIRED 10-DAY DETOX CLEANSE RECIPES AND FITNESS FOR SUPER BUSY PEOPLE

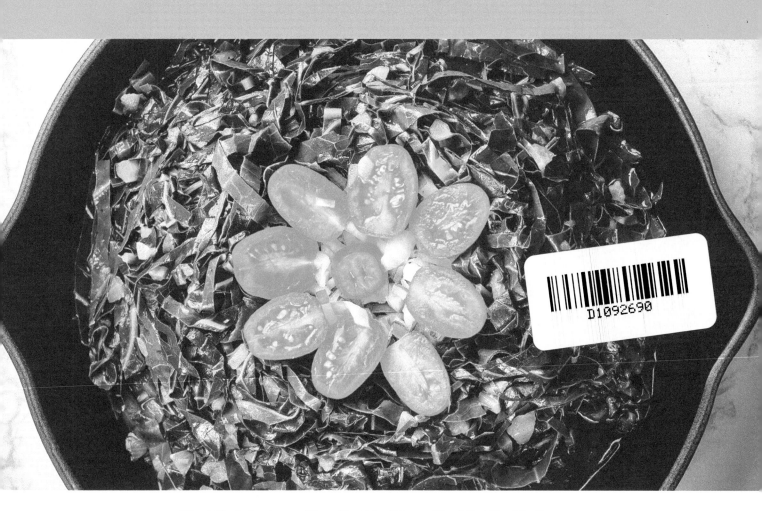

DENA DODD PERRY

Interior Graphics/Art Credit:
Smart Pixel Studio

Balboa Press books may be ordered through booksellers or by contacting:

Balboa Press
A Division of Hay House
1663 Liberty Drive
Bloomington, IN 47403
www.balboapress.com
1 (877) 407-4847

Library of Congress Control Number: 2018909654

ISBN: 978-1-9822-0251-4 (sc)
ISBN: 978-1-9822-0250-7 (e)

Print information available on the last page.

Balboa Press rev. date: 03/13/2019

BALBOA.
PRESS
A DIVISION OF HAY HOUSE

DETOXELICIOUS

EASY SOUL FOOD INSPIRED 10-DAY DETOX CLEANSE
RECIPES AND FITNESS FOR SUPER BUSY PEOPLE

What better way for my fellow Estrogen Warriors to take control. The time is now. Refresh... Reboot...Renew. Try it... the Orenda cleanse. Your body will thank you.

—**Sharon Dodd- Kimmey**, *M.D., Forensics Psychiatrist Medical Director Huron Valley Consultation Center*

As a board certified internist and specialist in women's health and anti-aging and regenerative medicine, I help women become self sustainably healthy through adopting a healthy lifestyle. Even the healthiest of my patients need help on that journey as our environment has become extremely toxic. To that end, periodic cleansing, targeting cellular detoxification has been my recommendation for decades. In the last 8 years, since sharing the detoxification products with my patients, I have seen more sustainable successes than ever before. The Clean Burn Shape products are the easiest, yet most sophisticated and scientifically supported nutritional support program I have ever used.

—**Vesna Skul**, *MD, FACP, Medical Director, Comprehensive Center for Women's Medicine*

I originally thought this detox cleanse would be difficult to incorporate into my busy schedule. However, with some planning up front, I found that it was easier than I anticipated. The increased energy is what brought me back for another cleanse!

—**Dominique Lash**, *MD, Physical Medicine and Rehabilitation*

Thank you to my loving family and friends for helping me share this detox lifestyle with all of you. I dedicate this book anyone who has decided to make a small change for the love of self. When you choose love, don't be shocked at how quickly the universe will move with you once you have decided to make a change. Surround yourself with family, good friends and the peacekeepers as the energy will sustain you in making lasting changes. We will get to where we need to be. Taking one day at a time, we strive to be the best versions of ourselves. We may hold on to old habits but we can make incremental lifestyle changes for better balance. To create better balance, use this detox guide to help you let go of what is not serving you well. You will find that the power of your own food-fitness experience will inspire others. Share your truth. Be patient. Be present. Be ready to do the work in order to learn, earn, give, and grow stronger. Take a deep inhale and exhale. Let's be "detoxelicious" together.

INTRODUCTION

This book is intended to be a powerful 10-day road map and self-help book to assist you on your detoxification journey. None of us is perfect. Written from the perspective of my experience with real people and integrative medical doctors, this detox book aims to make your time in the kitchen worth it because the food-fitness journey can be detoxifying AND delicious. All of the food is designed to be dairy-free, sugar-free, grain-free and plant-based, direct from mother nature. It's an easy, soul-food and fitness-inspired 10-Day detox cleanse for super busy people. I hope you'll share this book with someone you love.

How is delicious defined in the context of detoxifying your body?

How do we create simple detoxifying treats for a cleanse, or simply when we want to give the body nutrient-rich foods from nature? How do we relieve ourselves of the worry about the time and cost of food preparation in the rapid-paced world we live in? This book will help you to solve these mysteries in a simple and concise way. Let's own our power today. Let's not only make a change but make a difference with our health outcomes.

"Detoxification" means ensuring that your entire body is functioning at an optimal, balanced level, including your: immune, circulatory, digestive, respiratory systems; organs, vessels, and connective tissue. When your system is in balance, you are regular every day! And don't we all want that? Most women over 40 are prone to occasional constipation, food sensitivities or allergies.

It's common, but we don't want it to progress further into a more serious autoimmune disease. When your body is back in balance: 1) it can prevent your body from infections and other health issues; 2) assist in increased metabolism; 3) help you to achieve better digestion; and 4) contribute to a more energetic sense of well-being. After all, your body was made to heal. You can maintain balance and heal yourself. When that does not occur, disease can develop. It can make a difference in your life when you start the re-balancing process sooner rather than later.

Balancing life can be challenging. Are you tired of trying trendy, fad diets? Are you interested in regaining your youthful vitality? Do you feel like crap? Not only will most people feel amazing and attain better results in your medical checkups, but you will discover your best "detoxelicious" foods.

So, let's make food that is simple, delicious and uncomplicated. I grew up in a southern kitchen. Honestly, there have been days when I threw down in the kitchen. I cooked ham hocks in my soups. I cooked lemon-pepper chicken with homemade mac and cheese and collard greens with a pop of corn bread in the big mama iron skillet. Like most modern parents, I've struggled too. There have been many days that I couldn't be the "perfect wife" and prepare a detailed meal plan for the week. I've stared in the refrigerator and looked for answers that even Google could not find. I've made breakfast foods for dinner for the kids. I've even made cheese quesadillas and put some frozen pizza in the oven and called it a day.

As I started to write this book, I conducted my own ad-hoc focus group detox research with my family and friends. Everyone wanted food to be delicious or the detox to be easy. And time and time again, everyone wanted my homemade lentil soup or my down-home collard greens" or my daughter's watermelon-strawberry "juju smoothie," just to name a few family favorites. Some relatives were relieved to know that plant-based foods like my collards can be made without meat and still taste delicious.

I told them that I was first exposed to a detox cleanse when my husband turned 40 in 2005. At the time, the detox cleanse topic seemed obscure, foreign and quite frankly too mind-blowingly complicated. Since my husband had lived a progressive lifestyle, his willingness to try a new fiber-based detox seemed natural. My ad-hoc focus group knew him, so each responded favorably to a smart guy having a detox cleanse and seeing real weight loss results.

There are a wide variety of "detox cleanses" available to the public. They range from cayenne-lemon water to Paleo to juice cleanses to scientifically researched cleanses from overseas. I waited 12 years to try my first detoxification with an exclusively cold-pressed juice cleanse. Talk about a painful gastrointestinal experiment. I remember my belly grumbling every evening and having hour-long conversations with my friend trying to find any glimmer of hope from words that would indicate that I could "end" the starvation right then and there. I'd finish the three-day pure juice cleanse, but then wanted to take a quick trip to Chick-Fil-A for a basket of waffle fries.

I began to feel badly both in mind and body, about my digression. I know heart disease and some types of fibroid tumors run in my family. It felt like I had committed a cardinal sin. I was forced to analyze why my body felt so bad. I needed to find a construct which would explain it. I needed a simpler way to think about food. After the ultimate rebuking of my engineering mind, I thought to categorize food based on the way it made me feel. And quite frankly, I felt dirty. So, let's talk about perceived "dirty foods."

"Dirty foods" can be defined as processed foods or food grown with pesticides. "Clean foods" are described as food derived from nature without added chemicals or modifications. I began to shift my awareness to foods that gave me energy to grow. My whole mindset began to shift to Mother Nature. Rather than gravitating towards easy, man-made, and potentially genetically altered foods, I changed my whole mindset. I started to focus on natural choices. This mindset shift towards nature was transformative for me. I began to feel excited about connecting to the original source of food as Mother Nature intended.

Our culture is inundated with doing more with fewer resources. Everyone is multitasking to achieve the best results with the least amount of time for highest perceived value at both work and play. With the onslaught of social media and constant introduction of new "tech" toys, we seem to living be living life under the proverbial gun, leaving us with little time to create a sense of connectedness to each other and the overall experience of good, nutritious food. We have expectations of what we think life should be –taking walks, playing with the dog, laughing with friends, hugging our children, strolling along the beach. We struggle to seek a fundamental aspect of life that is simple. So, let's get back to basics and reset our bodies and our food. Let's do it "detoxeliciously."

TOP 14 FUNNY REASONS WHY YOU MIGHT WANT TO DO DETOX CLEANSE: ;-)

I am always having conversations with myself about food. Is this good? Is this bad? Can you relate? Well, here are just some funny food thoughts over the years. The purpose of this is to bring awareness to my food thoughts and break the habitual food cycle. Our thoughts about losing weight can be overwhelming or humorous. Today, we chose humorous. We also want to break the cycle of overeating. This is designed to make you laugh a bit in the process as it was written by both me and my sister, Shane Dodd, MD, psychiatrist. We like to poke fun at ourselves in an effort to not take ourselves too seriously. I am sharing my funny food journey with you to kick off your educational detox journey. Enjoy and have a good chuckle before you review the health statistics in the United States as of 2018.

I KNOW I NEED TO DETOX WHEN:

- The only ones that I miss in my life are a few doughnuts.
- I thought of bringing a giant spoon to the Super Bowl.
- I step on a scale, it reads, "to be continued."
- I've lost control of my eating and am at risk for tri-abetes.
- I realize I've picked up a few pounds and feel like I should use diet soap when in the shower.
- My holiday eating got so out of control that I wondered if my blood type was ketchup.
- I get the feeling that food trucks are following me around town.
- I've picked up a few pounds and feel that my own portraits will fall off of the wall.
- I flirt more with food than with men.
- I read nutritional labels on the cookie box and look for the, "What if I ate the whole damn box?" section.
- Everyone else is toxic but me.
- I have low energy, high stress levels and trouble sleeping with trash bags under my eyes.
- I have brain fog then..forgot I had brain fog.
- I have skin that looks like chocolate covered almond popsicles after applying my foundation.

WHY DETOX?

Detoxification is the process of getting rid of toxins. Generally speaking, we naturally eliminate toxins through our sweat, urine or bowel movements. However, our toxic load builds up over time. We need help from a good combination detox cleanse. I personally have seen the transformation of the quality of life for people who regularly detox two to four times a year. The primary principle focuses on giving your essential filter organs a break. Your filter organs include your liver, kidneys and pancreas. This detox cleanse also works to reduce some level of inflammation. Inflammation simply makes us more prone to a multitude of diseases, and can lead to complicated autoimmune diseases down the road. We know now from top nutritionists that good food leads to good health. Traditional western medicine is reactionary with an emphasis on making a sick person well again. The detox process focuses on preventative measures to improve, not necessarily cure, people's health. The goal is to make your detox delicious!

Here are some top baseline health statistics for women, specifically based on presentation data from the Women's Health Research Institute at Northwestern University.

Cardiology – Heart disease is the No. 1 killer of women worldwide, taking more lives than all forms of cancer combine; yet only 27% of participants in cardiovascular clinical trials are female. Women have a higher risk of stroke compared to men of same age. The data presented is from the 55- and 65-year old age groups (21% for women and 17% for men). The risk drops slightly in both groups as age increases, but remains elevated for females.

Immunology – Women are three times more likely to develop an autoimmune disorder than men. Women are four times more likely to develop tissue-hardening scleroderma than men. About 80% of your immune system lives in your gastrointestinal tract and probiotics can help regulate it according to the Institute of Health Sciences. Approximately 500 different species of bacteria live inside you. Moreover, eighty-five percent of breast cancer occurs in women who have no family history of breast cancer based on data from the National Institute of Environmental Health Services.

Dermatology – The majority of dermatological research uses male foreskin. Yes, I said it. Only 4% of studies report using female cells. Rosacea affects women three times more often than men.

Mental Health – Women are twice as likely to suffer from depression than men. Women have a 31% lifetime risk of developing an anxiety disorder compared to 19% for men.

Neurology – In the United States, two-thirds of individuals with Alzheimer's disease over the age of 65 are women (3.4 million). Women with Alzheimer's disease have a greater rate of cognitive decline than men.

So, what if it were possible to be preventive and proactive with our own health? Heart disease and fibroid tumors run in my family's medical history. For this book and for good reason, I canvassed and tried three different detox cleanses: a nutraceutical medical (MD) formulated cleanse; a famous protein-based cleanse with shakes; and a cold-pressed juice cleanse. I've never felt better or more alive than when I cut out the carbohydrates, sugar, grains, dairy, meat and bananas with the nutraceutical MD formulated cleanse. Essentially, the protein-based cleanse jacked up my cholesterol and the cold-pressed juice cleanse gave me an intense headache. In summary, going with a plant-based meal high in fiber is of greater benefit to you in the long run against illnesses like heart disease and cancer. This detox cleanse that I recommend is high in fiber and powerful antioxidant super foods to help you achieve better health outcomes. It's a game changer. See my personal experience assessment chart displaying opportunity size versus ease of use.

What do we know to be self-evident in society, health wise? Heart Disease is the No. 1 killer and cancer seems is more prevalent than ever. When we were little, you may have known only 1 in 100 persons with cancer. One out of every three people in the United States will be diagnosed with cancer according to latest statistics from the American Cancer Society (Source: Cancer.gov 2013-2015). We might even hear a friend or member has cancer and we ask, "oh what kind?" As a point of reference, doctors are keenly trained to react to diseases and their symptoms but not many are trained on the nutrition and its relative role to improving our health outcomes as almost all cancer patients must visit with a nutritionist after treatments. In summary, the overall cancer death rate has declined while the number of cancer survivors has increased.

Toxins and fat cells are not mutually exclusive. Generally speaking, toxins are stored in the fat cells. The fat cells feed off of sugars and synthetic chemicals received from the environment. If we dissolve the sugar in the liver that feeds the toxins, then we can possibly get rid of the toxic load at the cellular level. Healthy cells that have fewer toxins create better health outcomes, according to most integrative doctors. The detox cleanse that I recommend most as a wellness influencer contains powerful antioxidants. It is a patented detox cleanse that has the super powerful antioxidant support of the aronia berry. The "clean" supplement has potassium hydrogen glucarate, peptizyme serrapeptase (SP). The synergies of these ingredients along with additional herbs and extracts give us more confidence that supplements may attach to toxins and then be released or excreted out of the body. This is not a claim to cure any disease but prominent functional doctors, like Dr. Vesna Skul, of the Comprehensive Center for Women's Medicine, have seen some promising results in her 18,000+ patient cases with improved health outcomes when using this detox cleanse.

Weight can be a trigger of heart disease. A dramatic rise in obesity in the past few decades has become a global health challenge. Let's further review the numbers. According to the United States Department of Health and Human Services, two-thirds of adults are overweight and over one-third are obese. How do we explain this sudden rise in obesity? Some argue that people in today's society value convenience and as a result, make poor diet choices which leans toward animal-based and synthetic food products. With the proliferation of fast food restaurants and convenient food packaging, many are making poor diet choices on the go. Many people feel too overworked to find time to exercise. These lifestyle choices have a great impact on the health of Americans, leading to weight gain and increasing their odds of contracting potentially life-threatening illnesses such as Type II diabetes, cancer, cardiovascular disease and chronic kidney disease. It is estimated that obesity leads up to 3.4 million deaths worldwide (Ng et al. 2011).

However, while sedentary lifestyle certainly plays a role in obesity, the rapid rise of this health epidemic has led to widespread studies investigating whether there are other root causes of obesity. After all, eating a healthy diet and working out should keep obesity and health problems at bay, right? What if there are other contributing factors that are adding to the obesity epidemic?

In their studies of weight gain in the last few decades, researchers have noticed that something is affecting the genetic makeup of those who are obese. Obesity is found in children, teens and adults alike. Even laboratory animals and city rats have been gaining weight! This suggests that diet and exercise may not be the only factors in the obesity epidemic. Are there also environmental triggers which could be altering people's metabolic processes? (Holtcamp, 2012). We are starting to see greater evidence that there could be more to blame than fast food and lack of physical activity. Toxic chemical exposure, in addition to poor diet and lack of exercise, is an additional factor in the obesity epidemic (Grens, 2015).

Being skinny is no guarantee of good health. Some skinny people are slim, but not fit, and they do not have healthy habits. It does not eliminate your risk from toxins. "One in four skinny people have pre-diabetes and can be metabolically obese. The implications of being "skinny fat" puts your body under a huge amount of pressure, including unseen added fat around your organs, high cholesterol and poor circulation," according to Australian-based expert scientist and regulatory manager at USANA Health Sciences, Sheila Zhou,

So, what can you do to combat toxins quickly and become healthier from the inside out? Practice better self-care. Take a superior, scientific detox cleanse that removes toxins at the cellular level; reduce your consumption of artificial sweeteners in your soft drinks; commit to strength training with weights to activate core muscles; add select Omega-3 rich foods like salmon and sardines; drink tea that lowers your cortisol levels after a stressful week; and get your rest. Don't eat after 7pm. Everyone loves a good night's sleep, but how many of us actually get the required seven to eight hours a night? It's been scientifically proven that sleep deprivation alters your metabolism and increases cravings for carbs and sugar, hence and increases our exposure to toxins. Remember, sugar enhances fat cells where the toxins live and grow.

As it turns out, there are toxic chemicals everywhere around us. We breathe them in, use them on our skin, and consume them along with our meals. In the last 100 years, toxicity levels have increased drastically with the rise of convenient fast food and processed packaged products. In fact, it seems that growth in the use of synthetic chemicals in the last century has dramatically changed the way that the human body functions (Mason, 2006). As the use of chemical substances in the making of food and lifestyle products has increased over a 100-year period, obesity levels have skyrocketed. Thus, we see a correlation between the level of synthetic chemicals in the environment, or **obesogens**, and the world-wide obesity epidemic. I call these synthetic chemicals, "hood rats. These hood rats (or obesogens) are environmental chemicals found in our everyday lives that disrupt the endocrine system and promote weight gain.

Our endocrine system is responsible for the development, growth, behavior and reproductive functions in our bodies. It is essential to good health as it keeps our body in balance and maintains proper growth and development. It functions as a communication network and secretes hormones that regulate tissues in the body to help control the reproductive functions, stress and energy levels, and the metabolic system. However, when exposed to toxic chemicals such as the obesogens, the body's development is disrupted.

Such disruptions can have many adverse effects on our bodies. Hood rats can alter the function of the endocrine system by mimicking or disrupting the hormones in the body. They act to modify the signals that hormones normally have in our bodies, which change how our organs and tissues act. As a result, the body becomes more susceptible to immune, neurological, metabolic, developmental and reproductive problems. This unknown cause and effect can tell us that "you are what you eat," and build a compelling case to eat organic as much as possible.

How Does the Immune System Work?

"Your immune system begins its job at the boundaries between your body and the outside world. There are good bacteria and a whole lot of bad bacteria. Our goal is to always reduce inflammation. Your immune system operates on the surface of your skin when toxins land on it. Likewise, when you breathe in toxins through your nose and lungs, the tiny hair inside your nose and the hair-like cilia inside your lungs act as a physical barrier to prevent the invaders from entering. At the same time your immune system creates a chemical barrier producing the mucus in your nose and lungs that entrap and neutralize many of the hood rats.

Your immune system has two-parts: Innate normal and adaptive complex. Your first and fastest and more immediate line of defense is the innate system. This is the more primitive part of your immune system, the part you have in common with plants, fungi, insects, etc.

Your innate normal immune system frequently works through reducing inflammation. Inflammation is the hot, fiery reaction our bodies make to fight off an infection. If you cut your finger, for example, the innate immune system works control the spread of harmful bacteria. A person may experience redness, swelling, heat and pain. This is the baseline level of defense: intruder means inflammation and it's the only formula they know."

In contrast, your adaptive complex immune system takes longer to kick into action. In fact, the adaptive develops over time because it reacts to tons of information about which intruders have threatened you and how best to attack them, slowly building "immune shield" to protect you from unwanted infections or cooties.

Why Obeseogens Are So Bad?

Obesogens act like hormones and can mimic naturally occurring hormones in the body causing overstimulation of the natural hormones, preventing them from functioning properly. They can disrupt the hormone estrogen (the female sex hormone), androgen (the male sex hormone), the thyroid hormone and can block these hormones from proper cellular response. They also alter the energy balance, metabolism, and change how the body responds to appetite.

Obesogens disrupt the hormones that regulate weight by binding to a cellular receptor and interfering with the cell's normal response. They promote fat storage by causing growth in the size of fat cells and the quantity of fat cells in our bodies. Thus, stem cells are converted into fat cells. Our fat cells are supposed to store energy and release it when our body needs it. When everything in the body functions normally, metabolism hormones are released properly. However, when we expose ourselves to extra environmental aggravators and stress, the fat cells do not release signals correctly. For example, they can prevent the release of the hormone leptin disrupting normal appetite and the feeling of fullness after and while eating.

The rise of obesity in recent decades can also be attributed to past toxin exposure. Our parent's exposure to toxic chemicals might have contributed to the rise in obesity in the subsequent generations. Recent research revealed that exposure to endocrine disruptive chemicals and obesogens can cause obesity in future generations. In studies, it was found that rats exposed to these toxic chemicals became obese in the second and the third generations. These findings have interesting implications about the vulnerability of humans to weight gain from toxic exposure (Grens, 2015). It is possible that if we expose ourselves to more and more obesogens now, future generations will keep getting fatter.

Healthy gut bacteria are essential for weight maintenance, healthy digestion, and proper metabolic function. Microbes digest the food we eat and dissolve harmful compounds that enter our bodies. Any disruptions in our gut bacteria can lead to weight gain and other health problems. Toxic obesogens disrupt the ecology of the gut by altering the flora in the lining of the gut.

Gut bacteria are affected through the consumption of pesticide-ridden produce, consumption of processed food and exposure to antibiotics. When we consume toxic foods that are foreign to the body's natural bacteria, the body raises its levels of stress response hormones to fight the toxins entering the gut. As a result, the stress hormone, cortisol, is elevated and the body becomes vulnerable to infections and weight gain. Cravings are intensified as satiety is affected when the gut microbes are out of balance. To get your gut balanced, try finding a high-quality probiotic supplement. I have taken Mega Spore and the Orenda Eaze. You can find Orenda Eaze on the denadodd.com website.

Eating dairy and meat that have been exposed to antibiotics and other toxins is especially harmful to the gut. When we ingest these animal products, we are essentially exposing our body to whatever obesogens the animal was exposed to. These toxic environmental chemicals are hard to avoid if you are not aware of where your products and food come from and what contents you are consuming.

Obesogens can enter our bodies in many ways:

- Consuming produce that contains pesticides and herbicides
- Eating processed foods that disrupt gut bacteria
- Eating foods in plastic packaging
- Eating canned foods
- Breathing polluted air
- Drinking water
- Eating natural hormones found in soy products
- Consuming hormones from dairy and meat
- Using plastic
- Exposure to vinyl
- Using harmful laundry products
- Any household and cleaning products
- Exposing the skin to certain beauty, makeup, and personal care products

Because we constantly use these products, our lives may be over-contaminated with toxins obesogens. Thus, it is more important to become more conscious of what we buy going forward and read labels more carefully.

Here are some of the most dangerous obesogens:

- **Monosodium glutamate (MSG).** MSG is used as a food additive to increase the flavor of food in restaurants, and in foods like canned soups.

- **High Fructose Corn Syrup (HFCS).** The body is not able to metabolize HFCS as it does sugar and other natural sweeteners. In animal studies, it has been found that animals that consumed HFCS gained a lot more weight than those who consumed regular sugar.

- **BPA.** This synthetic hormone tricks the body to imitate the estrogen hormone and has been linked to insulin resistance, reproductive problems, cancers, obesity, early puberty and heart disease. BPA can be found in can lining and polycarbonate plastics.

- **Pesticides.** Thousands of pesticides hide in everyday produce and can be avoided by shopping organic.

- **Artificial Sweeteners.** These toxins are found in diet soda and promote appetite and weight gain. Artificial sweeteners are also known to disrupt healthy gut bacteria.

- **Tributyltin (TBT).** TBT binds to cellular receptors of stem cells and causes them to transform into fat cells instead of bone cells. In studies, these effects of TBT have been proven to occur pre-birth thereby interfering with the normal development of the fetus. TBT can be found in flame-retardants, certain paints and even in pesticides.

- **Polybrominated diphenylethers (PDBEs).** These flame retardants are found in electronics, building material, plastics, foam, cars, and furniture

- **Antibiotics.** Antibiotics negatively affect healthy gut bacteria and should be avoided unless prescribed by a medical doctor.

- **Arsenic.** Exposure to arsenic has been linked to increased diabetes. Specifically, arsenic interferes with the ability of the pancreas to regulate insulin.

- **PFOA.** This obesogen can be found on microwave popcorn bags and in nonstick cookware coatings.

- **Di(2-ethylhexyl) phthalate (DEHP)** is widely used in consumer food packaging, and polyvinyl chloride (PVC) medical devices. It is also found in some children's products.

- **Phytoestrogens.** Phytoestrogens are naturally occurring hormone-like substances from plants and they can mimic estrogen activity. They can be found in soy products. Other preservatives, like parabens,in beauty products can mimic estrogens too.

Directly ingesting obesogens through fruits and vegetables can be one of the fastest ways to increase toxicity levels in the body. Due to the high content of pesticides in some produce, we are gaining weight slowly even if we think we are eating a healthy diet. The good news is that toxin levels can be significantly reduced if these obesogen-prone foods are avoided. These foods have the highest amounts of pesticides and obesogens. It's our Dirty Dozen list for the grocery store is listed below.

- Apples
- Pears
- Strawberries
- Blueberries
- Grapes
- Peaches
- Nectarines
- Potatoes
- Lettuce
- Celery
- Tomatoes
- Cucumbers
- Bell peppers

Buying these items organic would significantly reduce your exposure to the toxic chemicals lurking in these foods.

Here is the game changer. The right detox cleanse can:

- Restore energy.
- Eliminate toxins at the cellular level level by using a cleanse that is rich with good fiber and has proprietary ions needed to attach to toxins and release them.
- Help balance the gut flora and reduces leakages which is what happens when the intestinal wall becomes irritated by sugars, prescription medications, alcohol, etc.
- Help with weight loss to reduce fat.
- Reduce inflammation and yeast infections.
- Stave off symptoms from certain diseases.

As shown are just a few of the detox cleanses I have taken in recent years. I evaluated them based on Ease of Use versus Opportunity Size for my own body. Each cleanse can be very beneficial to those who do not have contraindications. There may be health benefits with increasing your intake of super food fiber and adding more plant-based foods in general to your diet. So, it's a food game changer for some people.

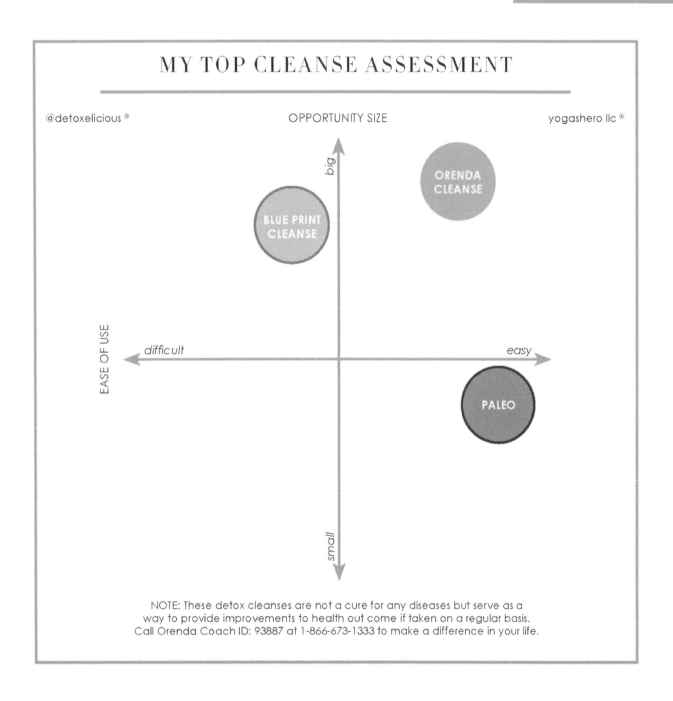

MY TOP CLEANSE ASSESSMENT

@detoxelicious ®   OPPORTUNITY SIZE   yogashero llc ®

big

ORENDA CLEANSE

BLUE PRINT CLEANSE

EASE OF USE

difficult   *easy*

PALEO

small

NOTE: These detox cleanses are not a cure for any diseases but serve as a
way to provide improvements to health out come if taken on a regular basis.
Call Orenda Coach ID: 93887 at 1-866-673-1333 to make a difference in your life.

Detox Is A Lifestyle

Detox is a continuous lifestyle! Here are some detox lifestyle suggestions and tips on how to avoid toxins. We must take an *inside-out* and an *outside-in* approach to have our detox cleanse work well for us. It's the "detoxelicious" way! Remember, the human body is made to heal. We detox through bowel movement, urine and sweat. Go to my website: denadodd.com

1. Find a cleanse that works best for you. A good detox cleanse can add real value to your lifestyle. Like the value of precious metals, each plant-based food has its respective value. Bronze has a different value than silver; silver has a different value than gold. Super foods are the gold-standard when it comes to nutritional value. I prefer to use super food supplements that are well-researched by functional medical doctors.

2. Buy and eat organic fiber-based plant foods as much as possible when choosing your fruits, vegetables and meats. Reduce your intake of simple sugars and complex carbohydrates. It is recommended that you detox three to four times a year.

3. Add strength training through weight lifting, or focus on the core abdominal training that exists within your yoga practice or Pilates fitness program. Never forget to drink plenty of water. Drink alkaline water when possible, which can be made at home. Use baking soda. Add 1/8 tablespoon of baking soda to an 8 oz. glass of water. Baking soda has a basic high alkaline content. When the baking soda powder mixes with the water, it increases the water's alkaline properties.

4. Detox your skin*, outside-in* with natural or chemically tested beauty and skin products and use natural cleaning products when possible. Not all chemicals are bad, so go with products that have a strong track record on better health outcomes.

5. Get your 7-8 hours of sleep every night. Rest is scientifically proven to increase the likelihood of making better food and fitness choices. And, in the long-run, it's better to commit to a holistic organic food, fitness and mindful lifestyle.

HOW TO BE DETOXELICIOUS

@detoxelicious ®   yogashero llc ®

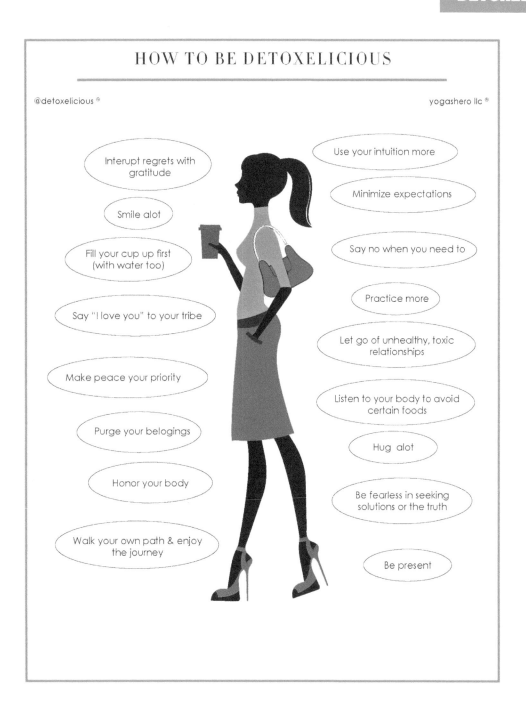

Interupt regrets with gratitude

Smile alot

Fill your cup up first (with water too)

Say "I love you" to your tribe

Make peace your priority

Purge your belogings

Honor your body

Walk your own path & enjoy the journey

Use your intuition more

Minimize expectations

Say no when you need to

Practice more

Let go of unhealthy, toxic relationships

Listen to your body to avoid certain foods

Hug alot

Be fearless in seeking solutions or the truth

Be present

What Are Some Outside-In Better Beauty Products We Can Use?

Body and personal care products contain thousands of colorants, additives, and toxic ingredients that qualify as 'hood rat' obesogens. These chemicals enter your blood after they are absorbed through your skin. Using organic and natural products is a great way to reduce your risk from toxins. Replacing multiple care products with coconut oil, lemon juice, organic oils and other natural ingredients can protect your health as well as save you money. Keeping harmful ingredients out of your skincare regimen is critical to maintaining your overall health. Using clean beauty products free of parabens, phthalates, and sulfates maximizes the benefits of keeping your skin glowing and radiant by preventing carcinogens, endocrine disruptors and other neurological toxins from entering your body.

So, what can we do about skin safer? I'm increasingly invested in energizing more women to feel empowered to make conscious decisions when choosing skincare and beauty products.

Why? A few reasons. First, we live in an age where information is readily available to us We know that our skin is our largest organ. Especially during the fall and winter months, we want to exfoliate and also moisturize safely. Did you know the beauty regulatory laws have not been changed since 1938? Many people do not know that companies are not required to disclose if sub-suppliers are shipping supply ingredients with pre-existing preservatives. Another point worth noting is that the word 'fragrance' in the beauty industry is a nebulous word that means anything can be in that synthetic bottle. A simple way to clean the body's skin is to use an organic sugar scrub or brush to get rid of dead skin cells on the skin's surface then use a natural oil on the body. Be mindful to avoid the face as some scrubs are irritating to the face and not the rest of the body.

DETOXELICIOUS BEAUTY SWAPS

@detoxelicious ®   yogashero llc ®

If using this...	Hook me up with this..	
Beauty and Body Care		
Mass Market Body Wash	Beauty Counter Body Wash	$24
	Dove Sensitive Bar	$8.50
Mass Market Shampoo	Beauty Counter Shampoo	$25
	True Botanicals	$34
Mass Market Conditioner	Beauty Counter Conditioner	$25
	Lavett & Chin Leave in Conditioner	32
Face Cleanser	Image Stem Cell Cleanser	$21
	Beauty Counter Charcoal Bar	$24
Foundation	BECCA Ultimate Coverage	$44
	Tarte Full Coverage	$39
	Beauty Counter Tint Skin	$41
Body Lotion	Beauty Counter Body Butter	$38
	Coconut Oil	MP
	Olive Oil	MP
Body Scrub	Beauty Counter Sugar Scrub	$40
	French Girl Scrub	$38
Nail Polish	Cuticle	$20
	Cote	$18
	Zoya	$20

Prices May Vary

What Are Some Outside-In Household Strategies We Can Use?

- **Avoid use of plastic.**

  For your storage needs, use washable canvas materials. Replace your plastic containers with glass and stainless-steel ones. Do not heat food in plastic containers as that process releases an extra dose of toxins. Skip the plastic wrap!

- **Avoid use of toxic cleaning materials**

  Use safe and eco-friendly household cleaning products and read labels to avoid the toxins. These are now sold at the mass-market stores. Avoid antibacterial products. Make your own cleaning products if possible!

- **Avoid synthetic fragrances**

  Use natural or organic essential oils like lemon, bergamot or lavender. Avoid artificial fresheners including bathroom sprays, home plug-ins, perfumes, dryer sheets, and other scents containing toxic chemicals.

- **Replace non-stick items**

  Avoid nonstick pots and pans are lined with toxic BPA and can enter your food when you cook. Replace with ceramic or glass cookware. Cook with full steel pots and pans.

Why Detox Your FOOD?

1. Glowing skin starts from the inside out. I'm almost 50 years old. I've tested a lot food and beauty products as a trained market researcher over the years and I'm here to share my own wisdom and observations. To support radiant skin, I drink lots of water and eat mostly organic whole foods. I also incorporate a source of Omega-3 in my meals with almonds, cod liver oil, chia seeds and the occasional nutritional shake. I notice that I have more of a glow when I do these things. Smoothies are also an easy, simple way to pack in fruits and veggies and get lots of fiber to keep you feeling full and reduce inflammation. Try the pre-frozen organic varieties from Costco, Target, Whole Foods or Trader Joe's and others. Then, add a non-dairy base like coconut milk, almond milk or filtered water and ice. Add ginger, turmeric, nut butter or avocado depending on your sassy versus saucy mood.

2. Any good healthy detox cleanse calls upon us to eat fruits and vegetables. Our goal is to keep the food irresistibly delicious. So, go for it and get your healthy drink on! Note: Please consult with your physician before starting any new nutritional program. For people with diabetes, you can use the advice from your nutritionist to eliminate any sugar spike-inducing foods like apples or carrots. Most people with diabetes do extremely well with the Orenda detox cleanse. My clients will text or call me with good blood lab results. But, everyone is different so always talk to your doctor and follow the cleanse instructions daily.

Eat organic fruits and vegetables.

Many conventionally grown fruits and vegetables are full of pesticides that contain obesogens. We have to avoid certain foods with some forethought and planning. Avoiding fruits and vegetables that are known to have high levels of pesticides will minimize your exposure to obesogens. If you cannot buy everything organic, it is important to know which fresh fruits and vegetables contain more pesticides than others. For instance, apples, pears, strawberries and celery contain lots of pesticides so buy these organic. Those fruits protected by a hard shell (like avocados, pineapple, and watermelon) are generally safer to eat in conventional version. Sweet potatoes, cauliflower, broccoli, and cabbage are also safer to eat conventionally.

Eat Grass-Fed meats.

If you eat meat, switch to grass-fed meat. Dairy products from grass-fed cows are also better for you than conventional dairy products.

Eliminate processed foods.

Avoid foods high in sugar, high fructose corn syrup, artificial sweeteners, and other toxins. Processed foods contain many foreign particles that your body does not recognize that can disrupt your gut bacteria. When your gut flora is out of balance, you are more susceptible to weight gain and metabolic dysfunction.

Avoid soy products.

Soy mimics naturally occurring hormone, estrogen, and can promote hormone-related health issues. Even if you don't directly eat soy, soy is hidden in many processed foods. Read labels carefully. If you cannot eliminate soy altogether, choose the organic and non-GMO products.

Avoid the use of antibiotics.

If you do not have a bacterial infection, antibiotics should not be used. Avoid animal products that are not organic, as that can also expose you to antibiotics.

Eat fiber.

Eat foods high in fiber and avoid refined flour, processed sugars and other processed items. This is important to regulate your gut bacteria.

Eat foods high in probiotics.

Probiotics are important in regulating gut bacteria and replenishing gut flora. Fermented foods are high in probiotics and include organic yogurts and kefir, miso soup, kimchi, kombucha and sauerkraut. See my recommendation for my favorite probiotic that comes with prebiotics and enzymes.

Lastly, to further eliminate toxins, a vegan-style detox four times a year is crucial to keeping your body strong. Reaching a healthy weight with a diet full of fiber and green vegetables can considerably reduce your exposure to endocrine-disrupting pesticides. Detoxing four times a year is the best way to cleanse your system of the unavoidable toxins we encounter each day. Eliminating obesogens from your lifestyle is not only important for yourself but also for your children and future generations. We have seen how dangerous toxic levels in our environment have gotten in the last 100 years and they are only rising. Fighting obesity begins through a more natural lifestyle and a nutritious diet.

DETOXELICIOUS FOOD TIPS

@detoxelicious ®   yogashero llc ®

If using this...	Hook me up with this..
Ingredients/Condiments	
Salt	Bragg's Amino Acid Coconut Amino Acid
Milk	Almond Milk Coconut Milk Rice Milk
Meat Broth or Cubes	Vegetable Broth
Dairy Probiotic	Coconut Kefir Coconut Yogurt Almond Yogurt Preserved Vinegar Pickles Miso Soup
Sugar	Coconut Nectar Stevia Drops, if needed

How Often Should You Detox?

It's important to detox your body regularly, perhaps three to four times a year. A regular vegan-style detox can help combat some of the harmful effects of obesogens. A 10-day detox diet should include lots of organic fruits and vegetables, and raw meals. While detoxing, eliminate all sugars, alcohol, processed foods, animal products, and grains. Green juices and smoothies should be consumed regularly to help the body oxygenate and release stored toxins. Furthermore, it takes your body less time to digest juice, so it can focus on getting rid of toxins.

Let's make it a goal to lose some weight. The goal is not to be skinny but to feel energetic. Because fat cells multiply through exposure to obesogens, the more fat cells or "lbs." you carry, the more they will keep multiplying. An important way to counteract this effect is to lose fat and reach a healthy weight. A healthier weight will help prevent health problems associated with obesity such as type II diabetes and cardiovascular issues. A healthy exercise program and a high fiber, safer diet should help you reach those goals.

THE DETOXELICIOUS WAY!

@detoxelicious ®   yogashero llc ®

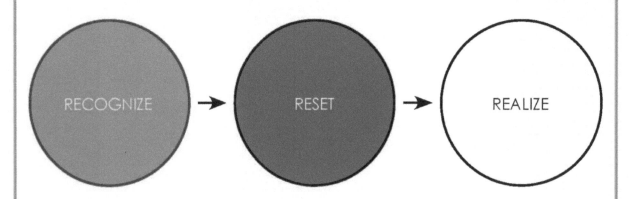

- IDENTIFY YOUR CHALLENGE

- GET A CHECK UP FROM YOUR DOCTOR

- RECOGNIZE YOU ONLY NEED A LITTLE PROTEIN TO FEEL HEALTHY AGAIN

- DETOXIFY AND RESET BY PICKING THE BEST CLEANSE FOR YOUR BODY

- RESTORE BALANCE BACK TO NUTRITION AND MAINTAIN DAILY BOWEL MOVEMENTS

- DO YOU!

- REALIZE YOUR RESULTS

- RECOMMIT TO SELF CARE EVERY 3 TO 6 MONTHS. PICK 2-3 DAYS A WEEK TO GO VEGAN

- BE GRATEFUL FOR YOUR BLESSINGS

Supplements Can Help You Detox

Probiotics

Take probiotic supplements if you cannot eat probiotic-rich foods on a regular basis. Probiotics are live bacteria that are good for your digestive system. They balance the good and bad bacteria in your body and keep your gut healthy. Probiotics also reduce abdominal fat, prevent obesity, and help keep you in shape.

Probiotic foods are cultured milk products and fermented foods. Sources of high-quality probiotic foods include live culture yogurt, kefir, buttermilk, sauerkraut, pickled vegetables, miso soup, raw cheese, and kimchi. Soy products like soy sauce, tempeh, and natto also contain good probiotics.

Some people cannot tolerate dairy products. If this is the case for you, make sure that you are eating fermented foods regularly. Eating fermented foods is one of the best ways to improve your gut flora. Fermented foods contain various strains of probiotics, are more easily digested and help balance stomach acid in the gut. These foods also help protect the stomach and intestinal lining.

Also, incorporating more fermented foods into your diet helps the body produce acetylcholine, which helps reduce constipation and improves bowel movements. Probiotic foods also assist in inhibiting the growth of pathogenic bacteria in your gut (Williams, 2016).

Prebiotics

Prebiotics are plant fibers that help promote good bacteria in your gut. They are like food for probiotics and they help keep the levels of probiotics in our bodies high. Taking prebiotic supplements is a great way to maintain the healthy digestive system.

Green Coffee Extract

Green coffee extract - from proprietary coffee varieties grown at a certain altitude - has been shown to help people lose weight. Green coffee extract helps to modulate the blood sugar levels in the liver and keeps them from rising rapidly.

Calcium-D-Glucarate

Calcium-D-Glucarate is a calcium salt derived from D-glucaric acid, which is found in many fruits and vegetables. This dietary supplement can aid the detoxification process by eliminating toxins (such as negative estrogen hormones) from the body. Since many obesogens cause the elevation of estrogen-like hormones in the body, this supplement can help fight obesity and other adverse health issues by reducing the body's toxic burden.

The food you eat can play an important role in altering the composition of your gut flora and promotes the natural detoxification process. If your diet is high in processed foods, toxins, and sugar, and is low in complete nutrients, you likely have a problem in your gut. Intestinal distress, cramps, bloating and other digestive issues may bother you on a daily basis.

Detox Yoga Fitness

I recommend that you exercise in a way that is sensible and healthy for your fitness level. No doubt that exercise will increase your metabolism and aid with circulation and digestion. The key systems of the body circulatory, digestive and lymph play a critical role in the elimination of wastes. The circulatory system pumps blood throughout the body, delivering oxygen to and carrying waste away from cells. The digestive system processes the food we eat and separates nutrients from wastes eliminating anything the body does not need. The lymphatic system collects intracellular fluid from throughout the body and transport it to the lymph nodes where anything harmful can be removed. The body releases toxins in one of three ways – poop, urine or sweat.

Any detox cleanse requires gentle exercises to stay happy and healthy. I've noticed that friends seem to enjoy yoga, walking or sauna the most while on their detox program. It's somehow easier on the mind and body when you stay active. Some people will experience headaches on Day 1 or Day 2 of their detox cleanse. This usually means they are not drinking enough water. So, drink plenty of water and do gentle fitness exercises like yoga to ease the pain of not having your usual food choices. You can take breaks but try to do your 10-day cleanse because it matters to your body and overall sense of well-being.

Yoga was intentionally developed to stretch, compress, push and pull every part of the body. It is particularly well-suited to keep the waste-removal departments of the body functioning well. Breath is a very important part of yoga. We unconsciously create bad habits in breathing that impede the lungs from inflating fully. High stress can lead to a tightened diaphragm, which then prevents a fully functioning exhalation process. Our bodies do not take as much oxygen when we inhale, and we end up not fully exhaling as much hazardous carbon dioxide as we should. Walking is easy on the back and allows you to get fresh air and new perspective in your environment. While the sauna allows you to sweat more than you normally would, and forces you to drink more water. In summary, pick and choose what you need from a fitness perspective on any given day of your detox. Make it fun and "detoxelicious!"

What Is The Detoxelicious Way?

I like to do this the detoxelicious way. Our bodies are complex health systems.. In order to get our bodies functioning at full throttle with good energy, it's better to take a no-dairy, no-meat, and no-sugar approach.

My "Detoxelicious Way" is comprised of mindfulness, yoga fitness and soul-food inspired food recipes. You'll also find:

Inspirational quotes for each day to achieve an easy, **mindfulness** approach to food and fitness. It provides you with a sense of compassion for our everyday struggles and challenges. And, this allows us to celebrate your successes too.

Fitness focus additive yoga poses for each day to stretch tense muscles, destress and gently detoxify our vital organs.

Food-based diet for each day is inspired by simple soul-food ingredients to comfort and support you during your cleanse... "Ain't nothing like a comfort food side option."

Question: *What detox cleanse do I currently use? As of 2018, I use the Orenda cleanse as recommended by my doctor but you can use the supplements you prefer. If interested, you can purchase the 10-Detox Orenda Cleanse in either Vanilla or Chocolate by calling Customer Service 1866-673-1333 with health sponsor code 93887. Ask your doctor before starting new food regimen. https://denadodd.com*

Each 10-Day Detox contains the following ingredients:

(30 UNITS) Clean – Clean prepackaged powder is formulated with the powerful antioxidant, aronia berry and other helpful alkaline-oriented dietary ingredients to rid the body of toxins.

(16 UNITS) Burn – Burn pill is included to dissolve sugars in the liver and thereby starve off some of your fat cells. Weight loss is usually an after effect. Results will vary from person to person

(16 UNITS) Shape – Shape powder is simply formulated with the top Super foods found around the world. It is loaded with Omega 3s, fiber and protein.

In addition to the recipes in this book, here are some good pre-made snack ideas that can be stored in your refrigerator at home or at work. You can find everything at your local grocery store. Remember, try to buy organic as much as possible. Check out labels at Target, Trader Joes, Whole Foods or Amazon. You've got some better options these days to help you along your detox journey.

SNACK ideas include carrots dipped in any hummus, celery, sliced cucumbers, bruschetta mix on cucumbers, salsa on celery boats, guacamole, apples with nut butter, and raw cherry tomatoes that can be popped in your mouth like candy!

Detoxelicious! Enjoy!

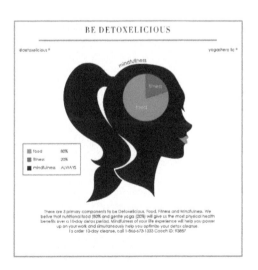

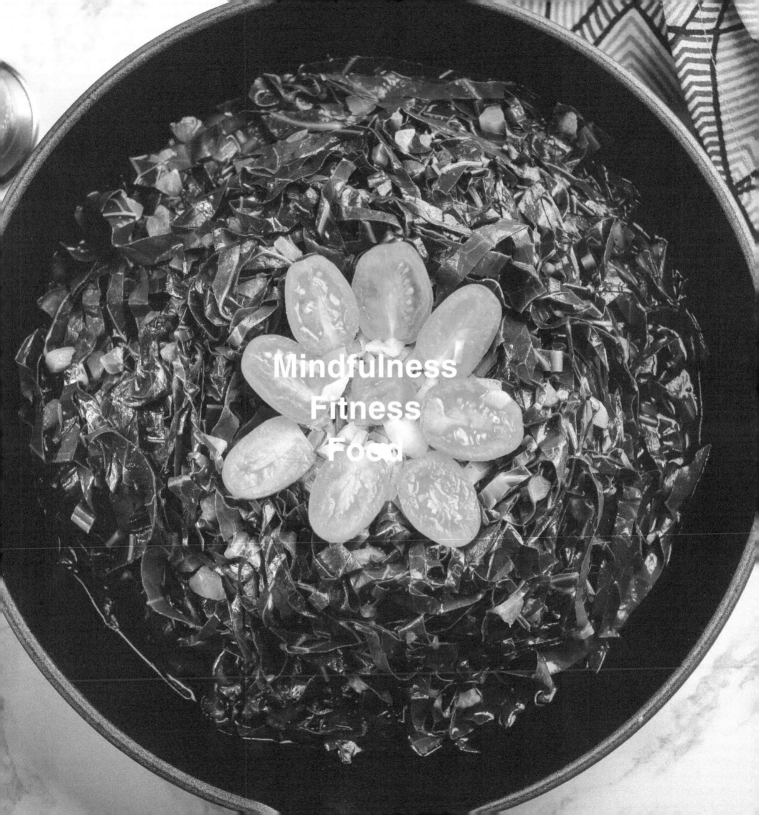

Mindfulness

Fitness

Food

MINDFULNESS

I believe the most important asset to maintain during and after your cleanse is a positive and healthy attitude. If during your cleanse, you eat something that is not "clean" or "healthy," don't beat yourself up about it. Don't give up. If you fall, then get yourself right back up. It will be helpful to carefully read through the foreword mindfulness quotes for each day. Feel free to write any thoughts or feelings you might have about your day. Reading positive affirmations and inspiring quotes will help you to clear your mind and become more aware of your senses and your mental and emotional spaces. As we become increasingly more aware of our thoughts, it focuses our attention in a more objective rather than a more judgmental manner. Reading positive materials helps to clear your mind of negative thoughts and feelings, and replace those negative thoughts with positive energy. Remember, we are not our thoughts; just observe them day by day. Your mindfulness principles will be provided daily in the recipe section of this book.

FITNESS YOGA

Here is a reminder that fitness can help to increase your metabolism, help in improving your circulation, help your digestive system function with more regularity, assist in improving muscle tone, reduce body fat (which can store toxins), help power up the perspiration which helps our body eliminate toxins more efficiently, and aid your respiratory system function and take in more oxygen which helps everything function better. Your muscles, skin and nervous system will be very happy that you've found a good detox cleanse.

Detox is a lifestyle. Even if you are very athletic, you might want to go easy on your body during your cleanse. Since you have simplified your daily intake and simplified the content of each meal, let your body adjust to this change. Also, people who are not used to exercising regularly may want to try a gentle approach to fitness. Yoga was developed to intrinsically stretch, gently compress, push and pull every part of the body. Try your best to refrain from strenuous exercises like running, kickboxing or cycling. Yoga is particularly well-suited to keep the waste-removal departments of the body functioning well. Remind yourself, hydrate around the clock and accept that good nutrition ultimately makes your body stronger. Your life is worth it!

Breath is very important part of yoga. We create bad habits in breathing that impede the lungs from inflating fully. Heightened stress leads to tightened diaphragm full exhalation. Yoga breathing involves taking longer, mindful breaths; inhaling through the nose instead of your mouth; keeping your chest still and letting the belly rise and fall. Aim to feel your breath moving throughout your whole body.

As stated earlier, yoga is an ideal exercise to complement your cleanse. Yoga can help raise your metabolism and stretch your muscles while contributing to your overall sense of well-being. If you are not familiar with yoga, start by taking a beginner's yoga or gentle yoga class. Restorative yoga is a good way to ease into things at a local yoga studio and learn how to execute the poses in proper alignment form.

My 10 favorite detox yoga poses are EASY. These 10 yoga poses encourage circulation of the blood via happy oxygen inhalation and lymph drainage from the feet and legs OR by squeezing the abdominal organs gently and stimulating digestion and elimination.

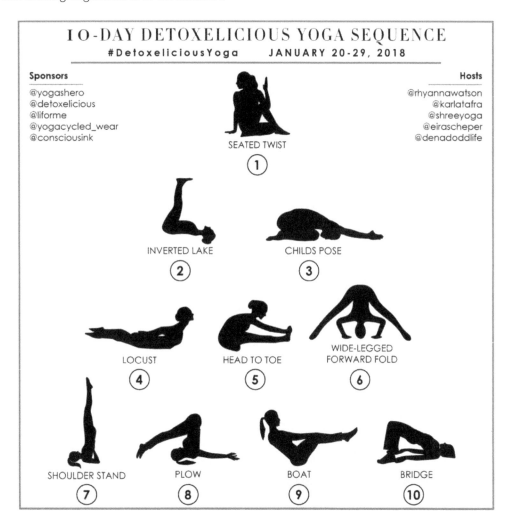

10-DAY DETOXELICIOUS YOGA SEQUENCE
#DetoxeliciousYoga   JANUARY 20-29, 2018

Sponsors
@yogashero
@detoxelicious
@liforme
@yogacycled_wear
@consciousink

Hosts
@rhyannawatson
@karlatafra
@shreeyoga
@eirascheper
@denadoddlife

SEATED TWIST
1

INVERTED LAKE
2

CHILDS POSE
3

LOCUST
4

HEAD TO TOE
5

WIDE-LEGGED FORWARD FOLD
6

SHOULDER STAND
7

PLOW
8

BOAT
9

BRIDGE
10

Detox Preparation: Breath of Fire

Key Actions: Rest easy on your back on a mat or the floor. Keep the mouth closed. Fill up the belly with air through the nose. And, quickly release the air through the nose. Start by holding you belly to feel the belly rise and fall. After a few practice breaths, quickly inhale and exhale for at least 20 to 30 cycles.

Benefits: Breath of Fire is a super detoxifier as it works to expel carbon dioxide. This is also one of the ways the body expels the excess acid. The exhalation of carbon dioxide represents the excretion of acids. So, this breathing technique helps to restore the body's pH balance. As a residual benefit, the Breath of Fire pose is also one the most effective ways to engage and strengthen your transverse abdominals, which act as a corset around the core of your torso.

Detoxelicious Day 1

Just Be Present. Maybe, being present is the present. Are you snubbing people you love by using your phone during dinner with family or friends? Are you truly watching for the weather forecast? Are you paying attention to what's going around you at work or at home? Take a moment each day to write down your thoughts unedited. Even though our feelings and emotions can grow turbulent, God's love for us remains steady. We must remember that we grow through what we go through. Then, take five minutes to meditate about your current circumstances. Think of your physical space and surroundings. Second, think of five senses. What are you touching, smelling, tasting, hearing or seeing? Third, reflect on your emotions, feelings and external images. Without judgment, create your own image of a page and make it a blank canvas. Begin to fill the page with your vision of happiness, physical body, work space and home space. Set limits for your phone usage. Your vision page is part of you. Your vision is created from your passion, purpose and power. Let's own this vision for the next ten days. Each day should begin with a healthy habit. All plant-based foods are part of your daily plan. You've got this, the "detoxelicious way!"

Daily Detox Pose 1: Seated Spinal Twist

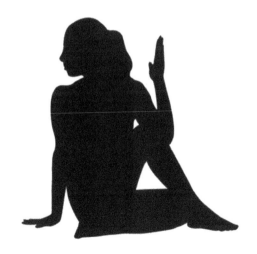

Key Actions: Sit down with knees pointed to the ceiling or sky. Swing left bent knee down adjacent to the floor with knee facing forward. Keep right knee bent with right foot just outside of the bent left knee. Inhale extend both arms overhead. Lower right hand behind your right sit bone. Place your left bent elbow outside the right bent knee. Root down on both sit bones. Rotate the mid-torso to right. Pull navel to back. Take your gaze towards the back wall over the right shoulder. Draw the crown of the head towards the ceiling. Hold for 5 breaths. Then, switch sides and hold for 5 breaths. Sanskrit name: Ardha Matseydrasana.

Benefit: Seated Spinal Twist promotes mild compression. This is one of the ways we can squeeze the abdominal (abs) muscles to stimulate digestion and elimination.

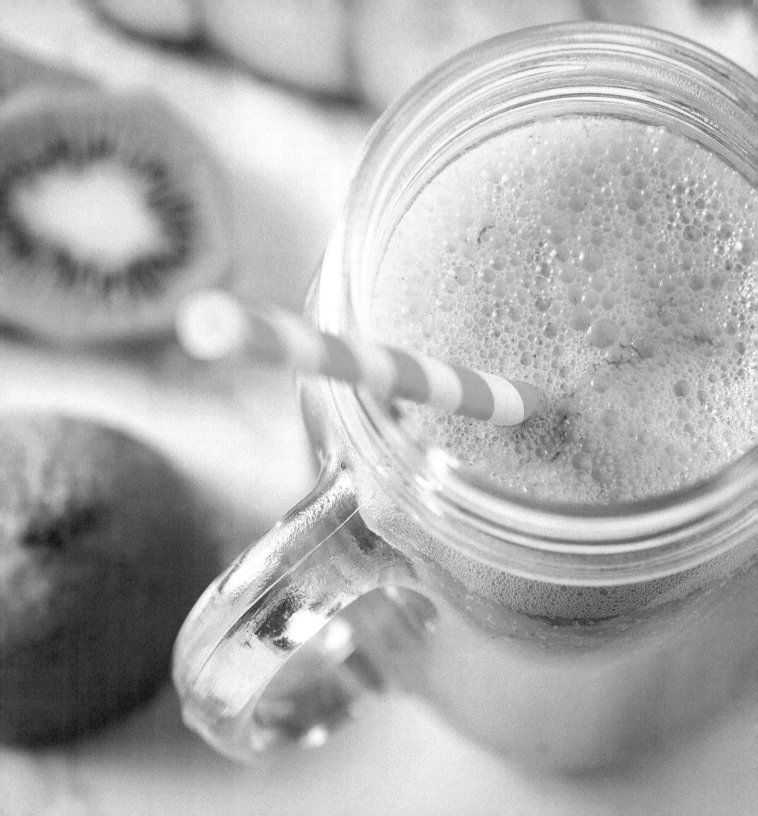

BREAKFAST

Bestie Green Smoothie

Serves 1 to 2 people.

INGREDIENTS

- 1 cup fresh spinach
- ½ of medium cucumber
- ½ cup chopped frozen pineapple
- ½ cup chopped frozen mango

INSTRUCTIONS

Total time: 2 to 3 minutes

Place spinach and cucumber and 1 cup filtered water in high speed blender. Puree until smooth. Add fruit and blend again.

RECIPE 411:

Be detoxelicious. My tip is to use at least one frozen fruit per smoothie and to fill up the blender with enough liquid so the liquid is above the level of solids. It's an easy trick when making smoothies regularly. It tastes so much more refreshing that way. You'll find that things go faster and faster once you discover which fruit and veggie combinations you prefer

Where are the BANANAS? Bananas have a higher glycemic index than allowed on mostdetox cleanses. So, we will not use them and give your organs a much-needed break from sugar overload. Feel free to substitute bananas with another fruit, like mangos or avocados.

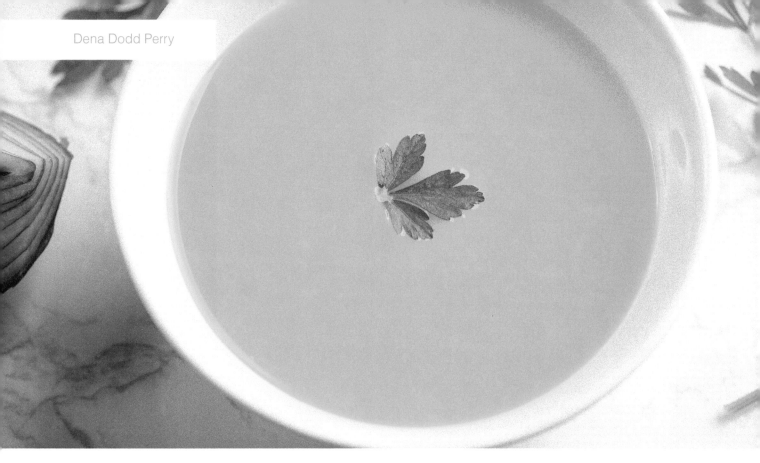

Dena Dodd Perry

LUNCH

DETOXELICIOUS
Easy Peasy Tomato Soup

Serves 6 to 7 people.

INGREDIENTS

- 6 cups organic vegetable broth
- 1/4 cup of frozen green peas, rinsed
- 14-ounce can of organic crushed tomatoes or equivalent
- 1 medium onion, chopped (or substitute frozen chopped onions)

- 1 cup chopped carrots
- 2 celery ribs with leaves, chopped
- 2 garlic cloves, minced
- ½ teaspoon dried marjoram
- 2 teaspoons dried basil
- ¼ ground coriander
- ½ teaspoon salt
- 1 tablespoon coconut liquid aminos
- ¼ teaspoon lemon pepper
- ¼ cup grated carrots

INSTRUCTIONS

Total time: 1-½ hours

In a large pot, combine the broth, peas, crushed tomatoes, onion, carrots, celery, garlic, marjoram, basil and coriander; bring to a boil. Reduce heat, cover and simmer for 1 hour or until peas are tender, stirring occasionally. Add salt and pepper; simmer 10 minutes longer.

Cool slightly. In small batches of 2 cups, puree in a high-speed blender; return to the pot. Heat for 5 minutes. Garnish with grated carrots.

RECIPE 411:

My favorite tip for anyone with diabetes in your family. Please go out and get a bottle of Coconut Amino Acid. It has a great flavor without the high glycemic index. Use the Coconut Amino Acid as your salt substitute. Also, eliminate any added high sugar fruits that adversely affect your sugar levels. You'll thank me later.

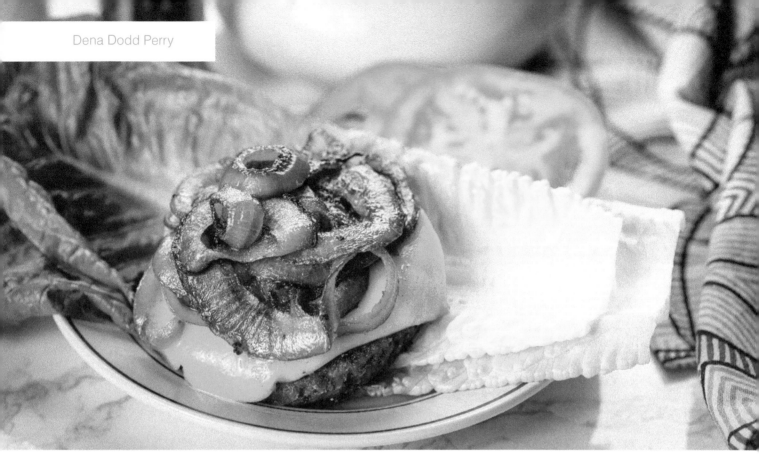

DINNER

DETOXELICIOUS
Beyond Cheeseburga! Cheeseburga!

Serves 1 to 2 people

INGREDIENTS

- 1/3 cup chopped onion
- Lemon pepper and seasonings salt to taste
- 2-Beyond Meat vegan patties, thawed
- Vegan American cheese slices

- 1 teaspoon vegan butter
- 2-3 lettuce leaves
- 2 slice tomatoes
- 1 tablespoon olive oil
- High-fructose-free barbecue sauce of your choice

INSTRUCTIONS

Total time: 20 to 30 minutes

Season chopped onions with lemon pepper and Lawry's seasoning salt. Heat a skillet over medium heat and sauté onions until translucent and set aside.

Season the thawed patties with salt and pepper. Heat a skillet over medium high heat and melt vegan butter in the pan.

Cook the patties for 3 minutes on one side then flip. Layer the cheese on the patties and cover the pan so the cheese evenly melts. Cook for 3 more minutes. Then, stack the vegan burgers with lettuce, sautéed onions, tomato and your favorite high-fructose free BBQ sauce.

RECIPE 411:

This burger recipe is a keeper. When I first tasted the Beyond Burger, it was love at first bite. I was truly smitten by the appearance of the pea protein patties bought with a real red mimicking tint. It's a true love affair. Every time I look at this finished meal, it says "eat me" with a gleam of grilled onions spilling off the side. So incredible, for real! Great for carnivores who want to swap for a healthier detoxelicious lifestyle!

Detoxelicious Day 2

COMPARISON IS A VIOLATION OF SELF

Social media has created a proliferation of distractions so difficult to avoid. I just figured out my own practice of awareness can help. I write quotes not only to share with you, but also to remind myself of what is important. Last week, I went down the black hole of social media and didn't go to bed until midnight because somehow, I ended up looking at other people's posts and comparing their life to mine. It was so non-yogic, an epic fail in my opinion. I felt horrible. I kept reminding myself that, "Comparison is the violation of the self." But sometimes, when you are in the abyss of self-pity, you fall into the depths of self-destruction. You derive a weird sort of comfort in going deeper into those negative thoughts. It's a sad state but the reality is that it happened. It's okay to be in this state of distorted self-reflection because you are not your thoughts. For this moment, you have the awareness to realize your thoughts are neither productive nor valid. You have shed light on your negative thoughts so let go of those thoughts. Be patient with yourself because you are doing your best. Now, let's move forward to where dreams are made. The lens in which you see your thoughts are clear. The outcome of this clarity with awareness will appear to unlock your mind to create definitively more beautiful and productive thoughts. Remember, your only competition is you and only you. So, when you see the sun rise again, know that you will be better than what you were yesterday.

Daily Detox Pose 2: Inverted Lake or Legs up the Wall

Key Actions: Place a bolster or rolled blanket mat width-wise along the wall. Place your bottom or sacrum onto the blanket so hips are slightly higher than the heart space. Extend the legs up the wall. Inhale and point; and exhale and flex the feet. Stay and hold position for 5-10 inhalation and exhalation cycles. Inhale through the nose and exhale through the mouth. Sanskrit name: Viparti Karani.

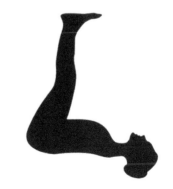

Benefits: This pose encourages blood to flow from the feet and legs to the rest of the body. Bathes the abdomen in fresh blood to stimulate the digestive organs. This soothes the nervous system, allowing your body to shift its attention from warding off stress to daily bodily functions.

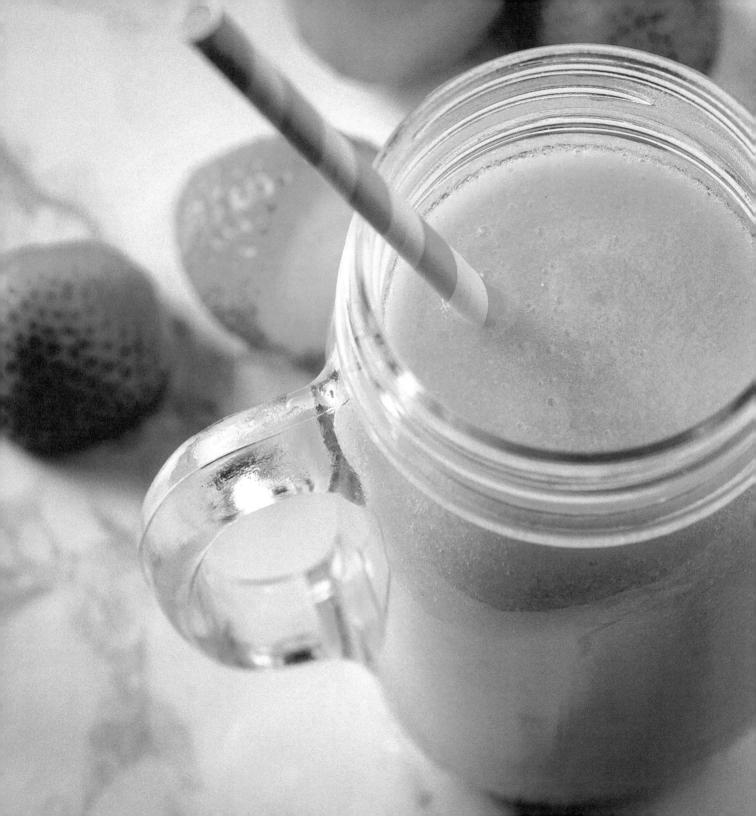

BREAKFAST

Berry Strawberry Smoothie

Serves 1 to 2 people.

INGREDIENTS

- 1 cup of watermelon pieces (or use mango or raspberries, if not in season)
- 3 ounces of frozen strawberries
- Juice of 1 lemon
- 1 teaspoon of stevia (optional)

INSTRUCTIONS

Total time: 4 to 7 minutes

Place strawberries and watermelon or equivalent into a blender. If not using watermelon, add 1 cup of filtered water then blend until smooth, if you do not have watermelon slices. Blend on low then high setting. Serve immediately.

RECIPE 411:

This is a personal favorite of mine and my "tween" daughter. We did a quick video of it on Facebook a few years ago. I can't tell you how many friends reposted their own versions. It's a joyful treat for everyone in the family or the busy working woman on the go. So, try to track down some juicy red watermelon to quench your thirst. Hooray for antioxidants!

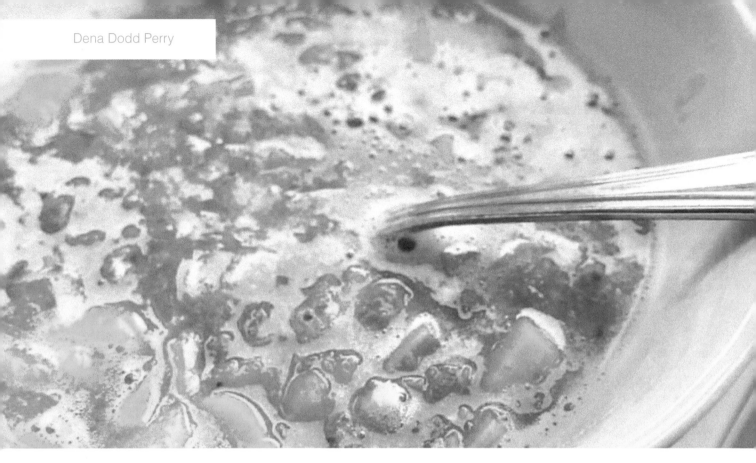

Day 2

LUNCH

Gentle Lentil Vegetable Soup

Serves 6 to 8 people (or one person for 5 days. Just refrigerate. Re-heat. Serve daily.)

INGREDIENTS

- 2 cups green or black lentils
- 1 tablespoon garlic salt
- 1 chopped green bell pepper
- 1 large chopped onion

- 2 tablespoons of olive oil
- 1 cup tomato sauce
- 2 bay leaves
- 1 teaspoon turmeric
- 2 teaspoons coriander
- 2 teaspoons lemon pepper
- 2 teaspoons basil or chopped fresh basil, if in season
- 1 tablespoon dried oregano
- 2 tablespoons coconut liquid aminos
- 1 quart of vegetable broth
- 1 package of mixed frozen vegetables

INSTRUCTIONS

Total time: 4 to 7 minutes

Rinse lentils, drain and set aside.

In a large soup pot, sauté the onions and green bell peppers with olive oil over medium heat. for about 10 minutes. Add all remaining ingredients, EXCEPT the bag of frozen vegetables cover with a lid. Cook for about 1 hour and stir occasionally. Add the frozen vegetables and continue to add a cup of filtered water if more liquid is needed.

RECIPE 411:

This is certainly a crowd pleaser. It's low in saturated fat, is cholesterol free, and high in iron, niacin, vitamin A and C. I've tried adding extra things to this recipe but I say if it ain't broke, then why fix it? It's a timeless soulful classic that good for your heart. And that, my friends, is something worth singing our praises. Amen sisters!!!

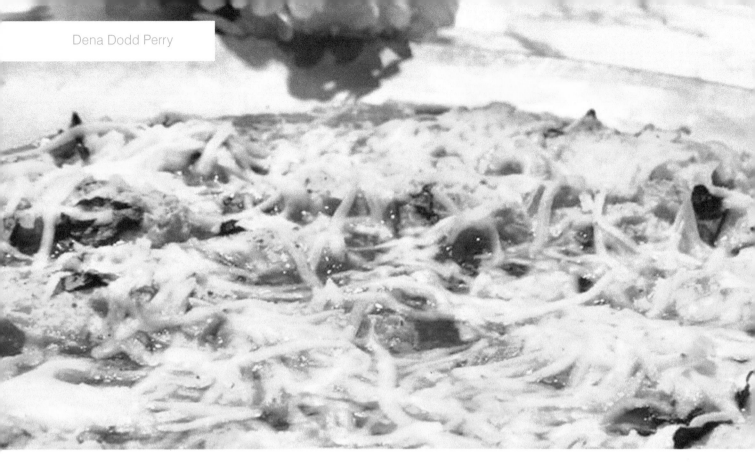

Day 2

DINNER

Vegan Barbecue Chicken Pizza

Serves 1 to 3 people

INGREDIENTS

- 1 cauliflower pizza crust (Trader Joe's has a good pre-made crust)
- 1 cup of frozen vegan chicken strips (Quorn or Beyond Meat versions both work)
- ½ cup high-fructose-free BBQ sauce
- 1 cup vegan mozzarella, shredded (available at Whole Foods or elsewhere)

- ¼ cup diced red onion
- 2 tablespoons chopped cilantro

INSTRUCTIONS

Preheat oven to 425F. Prepare cauliflower pizza crust as directed below. Combine the chicken and the barbecue sauce, top the pizza with the mixture, then sprinkle mozzarella and red onion and bake until the cheese is bubbling, about 10-15 minutes depending on your oven. Garnish with cilantro right away and serve.

Cauliflower Pizza Crust Recipe:

- 1 package of frozen cauliflower rice from your grocer
- ¼ cup egg whites
- ½ cup Parmesan cheese, vegan cheese preferred
- 1 teaspoon Italian seasoning
- 1 teaspoon of garlic salt
- ½ teaspoon of pepper

Thaw cauliflower rice and place cauliflower on a towel and squeeze any excess water from the rice mixture. In a medium bowl, mix cauliflower, egg whites, parmesan, Italian seasoning, salt and pepper. Press the mixture into a baking pizza round sheet or use parchment paper. Bake at 425F degree oven until golden brown usually about 15-20 minutes.

RECIPE 411:

Cauliflower is the queen mother of all vegan pizza crusts. Let's give it some dap. Once you try this, you'll likely consider making it again and again because it's so easy to prepare. I've used this with egg substitutes with little success so I wanted to reduce the fat and allow you to use egg whites for now. Using garbanzo bean flour, water and olive oil in equal portions as an egg substitute may work for you, if you are strict vegan. Try it the cauli-way today! Love you!

Detoxelicious Day 3

LIVE FORWARD.What are you still holding on to that isn't helping you? Let go of anything that does not serve you. Get rid of clutter. Release attachment to money, possessions, title, and yes, even people. Connect with our universal God. In order to receive abundant blessings, you must let go of the past to make way for the future. Many people do not know what letting go of past really means. They might be stuck in believing, "but they hurt me." We must forgive in order to remove the trashy baggage and make way for healthy choices in people, places and things. It's through forgiveness that we allow our self-love to shine brighter! We must have faith and live forward knowing that there are better days ahead.

Daily Detox Pose 3: Child's Pose

Key Actions: Face down. Pull your toes together and knees apart. Allow your chest and forehead to shift down towards your mat. Extend the arms overhead with fingers pointed forward. Breathe for 10 inhalation-exhalation cycles. Inhale through the nose and exhale through the mouth. Sanskrit: Balasana

Benefits: Child's pose, is in my opinion, the most supportive yoga pose. It helps to stretch the hips, thighs, and ankles while reducing stress and fatigue. When you reach the arms overhead, the pose gently stretches the muscles in the low back. If you have bad knees, I recommend you fold a blanket or sofa throw and place it inside the knee creases. This relaxes any tension surrounding the knees. See introduction yoga chart in the yoga fitness portion of this book.

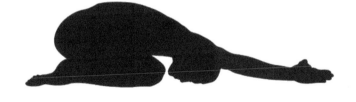

BREAKFAST

Orange-You Happy Smoothie

Serves 2 people.

INGREDIENTS

- 1 cup of unsweetened vanilla almond or coconut milk
- 2 oranges, peeled and cut in chunks
- 1 banana or avocado
- 4 ice cubes
- ¼ seedless cucumber
- Juice of ½ lemon

INSTRUCTIONS

Total time: 5 minutes

Place all ingredients inside a high-speed blender. Blend all ingredients for about 1 minute or until smooth. Pour into glasses and enjoy.

Day 3

LUNCH

Mediterranean Salad

Serves 2 to 3 people.

INGREDIENTS

- 4 cups torn romaine lettuce
- ½ cup of sliced cucumber
- ¼ cup quartered cherry tomatoes
- ¼ small red onion, thinly sliced
- ¼ cup julienned roasted sweet red peppers
- 4 pitted Greek olives, halved

DRESSING:

- ¼ cup red wine vinegar
- 1 minced garlic clove
- 1 teaspoon Italian seasoning
- ¼ teaspoon of coconut liquid aminos
- Juice from ½ lemon
- ¼ teaspoon each salt and pepper

INSTRUCTIONS

In a medium to large salad bowl, combine salad ingredients. In a jar with a tight-fitting lid, combine the remaining dressing ingredients; shake well. Drizzle some over the salad and reserve remaining dressing for another salad. Serve immediately.

RECIPE 411:

The recipe for the dressing is enough dressing in terms of quantity to use for the week during your detox cleanse. Please store in a steel or glass container from any large retailer. Store in the refrigerator and try to use within 5-7 days. Also, shown here are many store-bought, dairy free salad dressing varieties you can use and explore. This is not an endorsement of any of these brands but just purchase the ones you like and have fun with your salads during your 10-day detox cleanse.

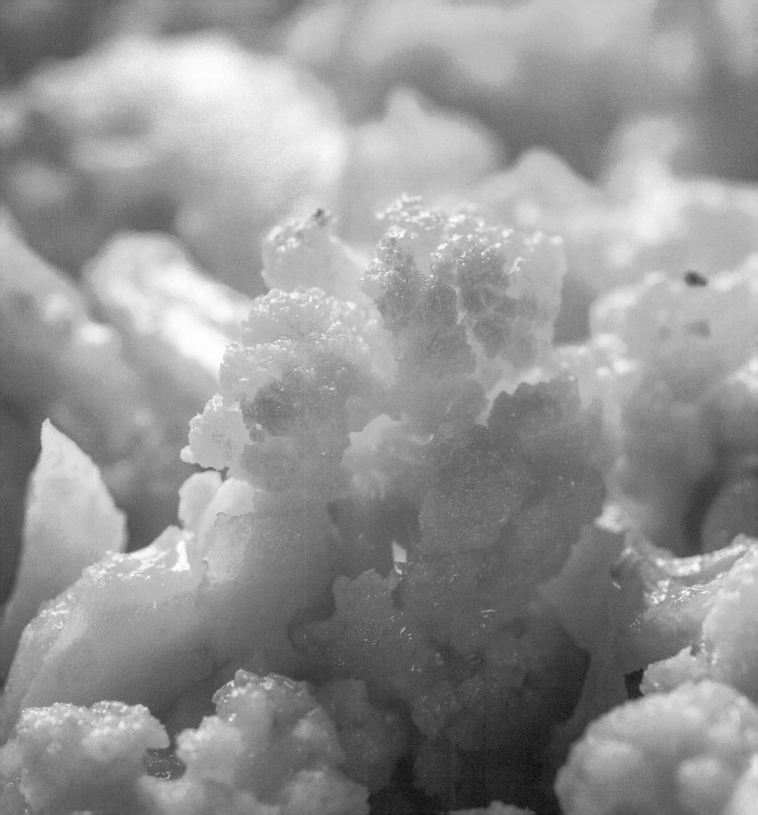

Day 3

DINNER

Hot Buffalo Cauliflower

Serves 4 people

INGREDIENTS

- Cooking spray
- 1/2 cup flour
- 1/2 cup water
- 1 teaspoon garlic powder
- 1/2 teaspoon salt
- 1/4 teaspoon black pepper
- 1 medium cauliflower, cut into bite-sized florets
- 2 tablespoons vegan butter, melted
- 2/3 cup Buffalo hot sauce
- Vegan Blue Cheese Dressing for dipping

  •

INSTRUCTIONS

1. Preheat oven to 450 degrees, spray a large steel cookie sheet with cooking spray and set aside

2. In a large bowl, whisk together flour, 1 cup water, garlic powder, salt and pepper. Add cauliflower florets and toss to coat. Distribute evenly onto cookie sheet and place in the oven. Bake for 12 minutes, and turnover florets at least one time. Remove from the oven.

3. In a separate bowl, stir together melted butter and buffalo hot sauce. Add baked cauliflower and toss to coat. Spread evenly onto cookie sheet. Place back in the oven and bake for 25-30 minutes or until crispy, turning over at least one time.

4. Remove from the oven and let sit for 10 minutes before serving.

5. Serve with your favorite "blue cheese" dressing and enjoy!

RECIPE 411:

Make sure you check out vegan blue cheese dressings that are available at your local grocer. It'll save you a little time. See our page with a picture of various hgih-fructose free and dairy-free options. And, my personal favorite baking vegan butter is made by Earth Balance. Most large grocers now have vegan butter near other refrigerated butters. Enjoy the flavorful heat in this one!

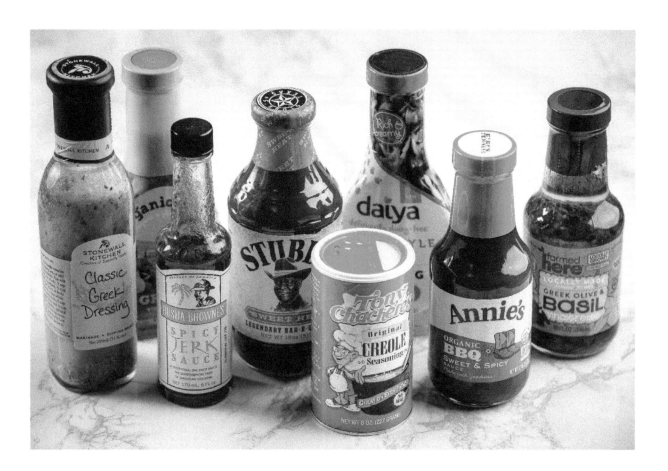

Detoxelicious Day 4

OWN YOUR POWER

You alone are all powerful because no one is you but you. Often times, we look to others for inspiration or to solve our problems. You are your own unique being with your own unique skills and talents. You have to recognize who you are. Are you a relationship builder? Are you loving? Are you influencing others? Are you good at getting things done? Are you a good listener? Are you a good talker, chef, writer or singer? Are you good with numbers? Use your skills. Own your power, be patient with yourself and seek more knowledge within your skill set. Get dressed up and go make that money. You are powerful. You are qualified. You are beautiful. You are confident. You are love. Remember these beautiful attributes as you walk through life. Quite frankly, if you reflect enough, you become your own source of light. Live in your own power but you have to do the work. Don't give up. Let's go.

Daily Detox Pose 4: Locust Pose

Lay flat onto the mat with your belly facing downward. Take an inhale. Lift the head, arms and legs off the mat giving extension of the entire back and firing up the glute muscles. Belly remains grounded. Note: Prefer to prep with lying on belly taking one hand and grabbing same side foot. Pull foot towards the sit bones. Alternate sides to stretch the quads first.

Sanskrit name: Salabasana.

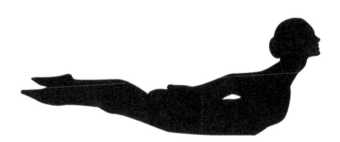

Benefit: Locust pose is designed to squeeze the abs and to experience an easy, supported chest opener. The shoulder blades become restored with continuous practice.

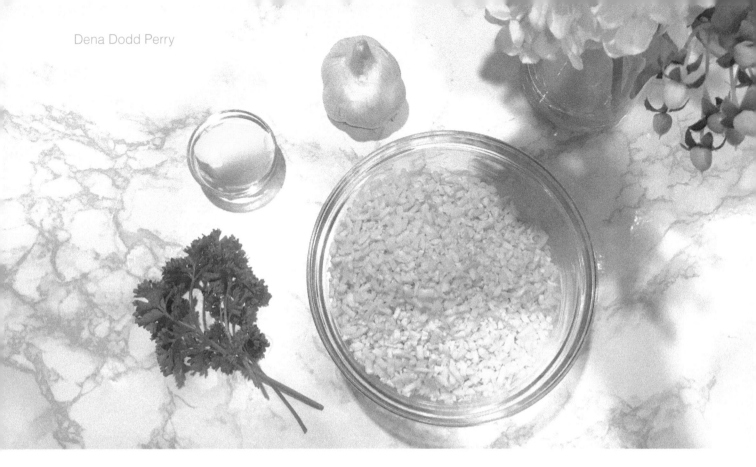

Dena Dodd Perry

Day 4

BREAKFAST

Cauliflower Garlic Grits

Serves 1 to 2 people

INGREDIENTS

- 1 cup of cauliflower rice (buy in the bag or make your own)
- 1 tablespoons olive oil
- ¼ cup vegetable broth
- 1 tablespoon vegan butter

- 1 teaspoon garlic powder
- 1 teaspoon of onion powder
- ¼ cup vegan cheddar cheese (optional)
- ¼ cup diced green onions

INSTRUCTIONS

Using a food processor with grater attachment, grate the cauliflower or shop for the prepackaged version of cauliflower rice. In a large skillet, heat on medium the olive oil and broth over medium heat and then add the cauliflower rice. Sauté 7-10 minutes until soft. Stir in butter, garlic, onion powder and cheese until all liquid has evaporated. Sprinkle with chopped green onions. Serve immediately.

RECIPE 411:

You will want your food to look gorgeous and delicious. This is a show stopper. Most Moms will take great pleasure knowing their cauliflower grits are really healthy. It's worth it to find the pre-packaged version of the cauliflower rice. Enjoy this deceivingly savory dish. Love you!

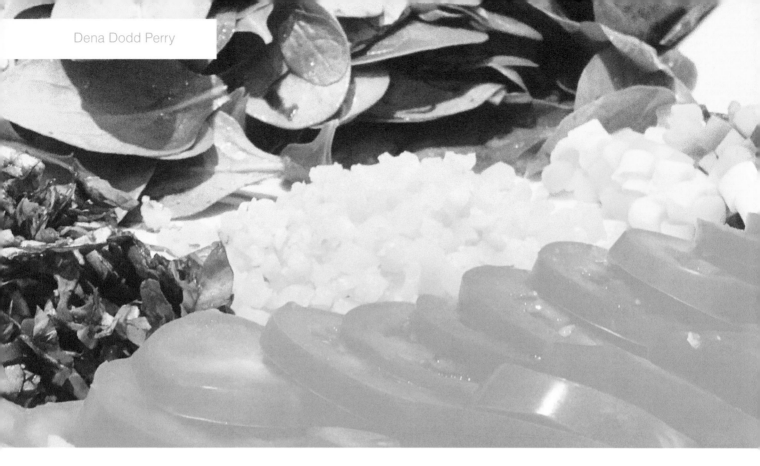

LUNCH

Southern Spinach Salad

Serves 4 people.

INGREDIENTS

- 4 pieces of cooked, vegan bacon, crumbled
- 8 cups fresh, washed organic baby spinach, dried really well
- 1 cup cherry tomatoes, halved
- 1 cup sliced cucumbers

- ½ red onion, sliced very thinly
- Warm vegan honey mustard dressing (store-bought)

INSTRUCTIONS

Place grill pan on burner and set to medium high. Grill up the vegan bacon 2-3 minutes per side. Place clean spinach in a large mixing bowl. Arrange crumbled bacon, tomatoes, cucumbers and onion on top of the greens. Gently drizzle with warm vegan honey mustard dressing or your favorite dressing. Toss gently then serve.

RECIPE 411:

I have a few favorite brands for vegan salad dressings. To shop for vegan honey mustard dressing, try common brands like Follow Your Heart, Annie's or Paul Newman's Organic Honey Mustard. Explore and have fun with the dairy-free, gluten-free brands. You never know what you'll find on your journey.

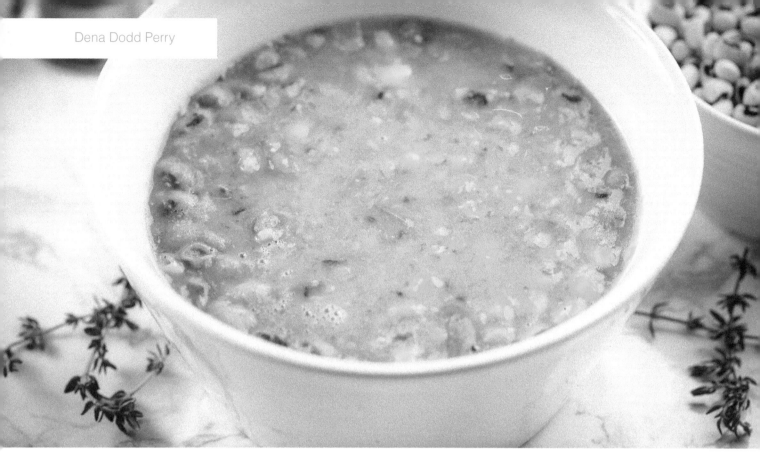

Day 4

DINNER

Hip-Hoppin' John Black-Eyed Peas

Serves 4 people as a one-dish meal.

INGREDIENTS

- 1 cup dried black-eyed peas
- 1 tablespoon vegetable oil
- 1 medium yellow onion, chopped
- 1 garlic clove, minced

- 2-1/2 cups vegetable broth
- 1 cup uncooked cauliflower rice
- 1 teaspoon crushed hot red pepper flakes
- 1 small green bell pepper, membranes removed, chopped
- 1 bay leaf
- 1 tablespoon chopped fresh thyme or 1 teaspoon dry thyme
- 1 tablespoon coconut liquid aminos
- ½ teaspoon salt
- ½ teaspoon red pepper seasoning

INSTRUCTIONS

Place peas in colander, rinse thoroughly with cold running water, picking through and discarding broken, damaged peas and any debris. In a large bowl, cover peas with 1 quart of water and soak overnight. Drain peas and discard water, transfer peas to colander and rinse with cold running water.

In a soup pot, cover soaked peas with 5 cups of fresh water. Bring to a boil; reduce heat to low. Simmer peas until tender yet still firm, about 40 minutes.

Meanwhile, in a large skillet, heat vegetable oil. Sauté the onion and garlic until golden brown for about 5-7 minutes. Add vegetable broth. Add sautéed onion mixture and remaining ingredients to pot with peas. Stir until mixed well. Cover tightly, cook over low heat until cauliflower rice and peas are tender, around 15 minutes. Discard bay leaf. Allow soup to sit and then serve.

RECIPE 411:

Many close friends complain that their black-eyed peas do not break down properly. I recommend you use the vegetable broth and coconut amino acid to help get the kind of smooth texture you want for your Hoppin' John recipe. Feel free to cook it a little longer, if you want your peas mushy like Grandma would make it. But, remember the yogic principle: too much of anything can be bad for us and can eliminate its nutritional value. Try this vegan method detoxeliciously.

Detoxelicious Day 5

BE YOUR OWN SHERO

Rock bottom has built more "sheroes" than privilege. First, let's start by interrupting our anxiety with gratitude for the future. We don't know what tomorrow may bring but we can always look ahead with hope. Second, let's see the beauty in all things. Maybe, one door closes for a better door to open. Third, recognize that it's the journey, not the destination that matters. One day, things will go in your favor, and then the next day, go awry. Like Martin Luther King, Jr. said, "If you can't fly then run, if you can't run then walk, if you can't walk then crawl, but whatever you do, you have to keep moving forward." Let's keep moving together in peace towards the finish line!

Daily Detox Pose 5: Head to Knee Pose.

Key Actions: Extend both legs forward flat on the mat. Bend left knee and place left foot onto right thigh. Inhale and extend both arms overhead towards the sky. Exhale and forward fold using a strap around the arch of the foot, or grab the right foot with your fingers. Hold for 5 inhalation/exhalation cycles. Sanskrit name: Janu Sirsasana.

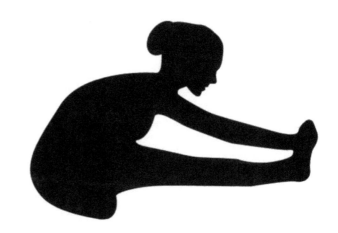

Benefit: The easy seated forward fold is designed to squeeze and gently compress the abs. It aids digestion and draws more blood to essential organs like kidneys, liver and pancreas.

BREAKFAST

Pineapple Coconut Smoothie

Serves 1 to 2 people.

INGREDIENTS

- 2 cup frozen pineapple chunks
- ¼ cup coconut flakes
- 1 cup coconut milk
- 1 small avocado
- Juice of ½ lemon

INSTRUCTIONS

Total time: 4 to 7 minutes

Place all ingredients inside a high-speed blender. Blend all ingredients for about 1 minutes until smooth. Add a little filtered water to thin, if desired. Pour into 2 glasses and drink up.

RECIPE 411:

This is an O.G. "original gangsta" recipe that is packed with super foods and good nutrients. In terms of a little trade secret, always add an avocado half, if you cannot bear the taste of grit in your smoothies. It's a smoothie pleaser, every time!

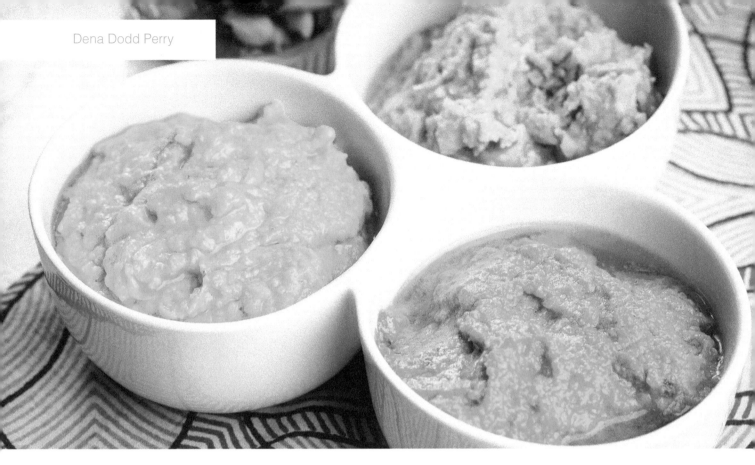

Day 5

LUNCH

Easy Green Peasy Hummus

Serves 2 to 4 people

INGREDIENTS

- 1 cup frozen green peas, defrosted, plus more for garnish
- 2 cups cooked or canned chickpeas
- 2 cloves peeled garlic

- 3 tablespoons extra virgin olive oil
- a pinch of salt and pepper and teaspoon coconut liquid aminos

INSTRUCTIONS

Combine all ingredients in a food processor until smooth.Serve with some peas on top and dip away! Use celery or carrots instead of crackers or chips.

RECIPE 411:

This is an easy recipe. You can make a protein-packed hummus snack from almost any vegetable including green, carrots and beets. So, let your creative groove thing go and try something new, fresh and exciting.

Day 5

DINNER

BBQ Chicken Fingers & Broccoli

INGREDIENTS

- 1 box of Ian's or Quorn chicken nuggets
- 1 frozen package of organic broccoli
- 1 high-fructose-free barbecue sauce

INSTRUCTIONS

1. Follow box instructions.
2. Boil about 1 cup of water and ½ cup of vegetable broth in a pot.
3. Once liquid is up to a boil, empty broccoli from its packaging. Boil for 5-7 minutes.
4. Stir. Do not overcook the broccoli. Drain and cool for 5 minutes.
5. Remove nuggets from the oven, then arrange nuggets, broccoli and barbecue sauce on your plate.

RECIPE 411:

Are you busy today? We know you are. Sometimes, you just don't have the time to throw down in the kitchen. This is just a quick recipe that you can share with the kids as well. We wanted to balance out homemade soul-food-inspired recipes with easy, everyday cooking for you and your family. Eat up.

Detoxelicious Day 6

BE UP FOR THE CHALLENGE

Look at your entire life's journey. Something that annoys you challenges you to be patient. Someone who abandons you challenges you to be independent. Something that angers you challenges you to be forgiving and compassionate. Something that has power over you challenges you to take your power back. Something you hate challenges you to love unconditionally. Something you fear challenges you to be courageous. Something you can't control is teaching you how to let go. We grow the most through overcoming our challenges. The challenge can be our greatest teacher.

Daily Detox Pose 6: Wide-Legged Forward Fold

Key Actions: Heart is above the head in this pose. Spread feet far apart along the mat. Point toes slightly inward and heels outward. Inhale the torso upward halfway lift. Exhale forward fold with the crown of the head facing the mat on the floor. This adduction forward bend is probably the safest, most accessible inversion in all of the yoga practice. Hold for 5 breaths. Sanskrit name: Prasarita Padottanasana.

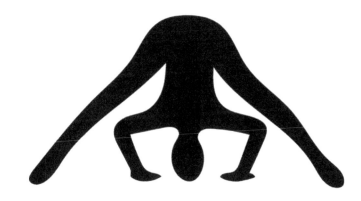

Benefit: Wide-legged forward fold stretches the muscles from the midsection to the adductors along the inner thighs. This will strengthen the hamstrings, calves, hips, low back and spine. It also encourages blood from the midsection the head.

BREAKFAST

Serves 1 to 2 people.

Protein Blueberry Smoothie

INGREDIENTS

- 2 tablespoons of chia seeds
- 1 cup unsweetened vanilla almond milk
- 1 cup frozen blueberries
- ½ avocado, peeled and scooped
- 2 dates

INSTRUCTIONS

Mix chia seeds with ½ cup of vanilla almond milk. Whisk until combined. Cover and chill in the refrigerator for 15 minutes.

Get mixture from refrigerator and put into blender with remaining almond milk. Add blueberries and avocado. Add filtered water until liquid level is the same eye level as the solid blueberries. Blend until smooth, about 1 minute.

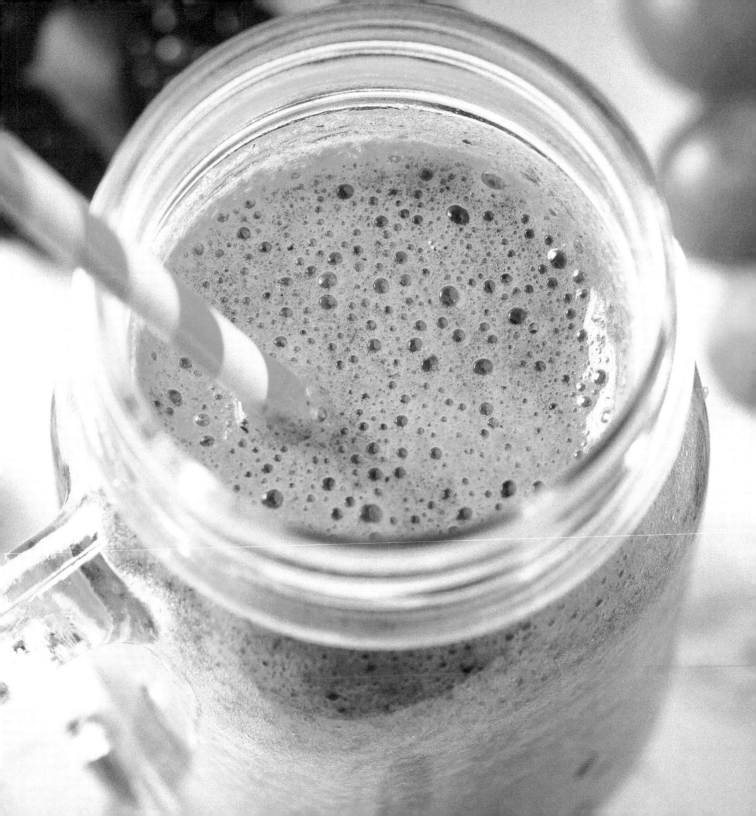

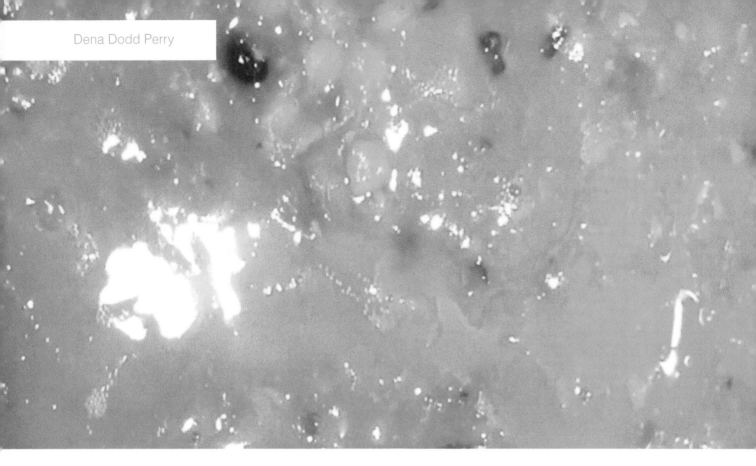

Day 6

LUNCH

African Fire Vegetarian Chili Serves 4 to 6 people.

INGREDIENTS

- 2 tablespoons extra-virgin olive oil
- 2 tablespoons coconut liquid aminos
- 1/2 large yellow onion, finely diced
- 1 cup diced carrot pieces
- 1/2 large red bell pepper, seeds and ribs removed, cut int small dice

- 2 cloves garlic, peeled and minced
- 3/4 teaspoon mild chili powder
- 1/2 teaspoon ground cumin
- 1/4 teaspoon freshly ground black pepper
- ¼ teaspoon curry powder (optional)
- 1/2 teaspoon dried thyme
- One 28-ounce can whole peeled tomatoes with their juice or 6 roma tomatoes
- 1/2 cup lentils rinsed and drained
- One 14-ounce can black beans, rinsed and drained
- One 14-ounce can kidney beans, rinsed and drained
- Big pinch coarse salt
- tablespoon tomato paste
- Shredded vegan cheese, chopped cilantro and scallions for garnish

INSTRUCTIONS

Heat the olive oil in a medium soup pot over medium heat. Add the coconut aminos, onion, carrot, bell pepper, garlic, chili powder, cumin, black pepper, curry powder and thyme. Cook, stirring, for 15 minutes, or until the vegetables are softened. Stir.

Turn the heat up to high, add the tomatoes and their juice, crushing them a bit with your wooden spoon, and bring to a boil. Reduce the heat to low and simmer for 40 minutes.

Add the lentils and beans. Fill one 14-ounce can with water and add it to the pot, along with the salt. Bring to a boil, lower the heat, and simmer for 40 minutes.

Stir in the tomato paste and cook for 20 more minutes, or until the lentils are soft and the flavors are melded.

RECIPE 411:

This is my fall and winter go-to meal for the family. The kids like to top this off with cheddar cheese, chopped scallions and plain Greek yogurt. Since this is a vegan "detoxelicious" book, we will avoid yogurt. Also, I like to use Roma tomatoes. The Roma tomato is less acidic and reduces the cooking time, but using canned tomatoes is fine. A good African stew is one that has a noticeable tomato presence with smooth exotic flavors. When you are finished and ready to serve this tasty chili, go with topping the chili off with chopped cilantro, scallions and vegan cheese or even a splash of hot sauce. Avoiding the diary will still make this stew very "detoxelicious" and help you achieve your heathy weight goals.

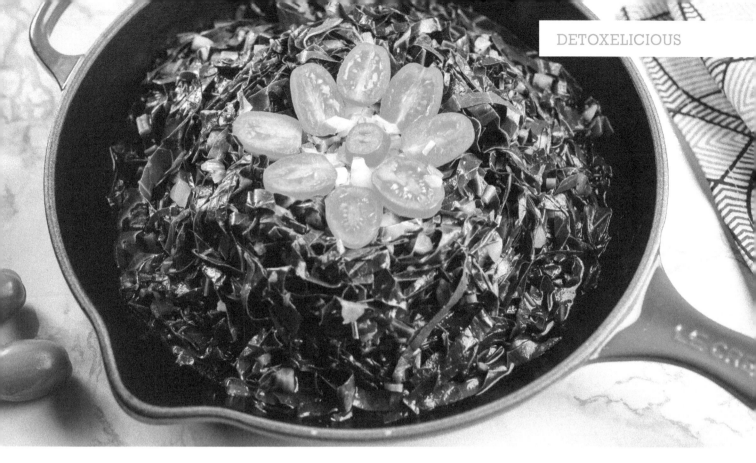

DINNER

Not-Yo-Mama's Collard Greens

Serves 4 to 6 people.

INGREDIENTS

- Three bunches of collard greens, soak in warm water, de-stemmed & cut
- 2 tablespoons olive oil or coconut oil
- 1 large chopped onion
- 1 teaspoon red pepper flakes
- 1 minced garlic clove or 1 teaspoon granulated garlic

- 2 tablespoon coconut liquid aminos
- 2 tablespoon balsamic vinegar
- 4 cups vegetable stock
- 2 tomatoes, chopped
- Garlic salt and pepper to taste.

INSTRUCTIONS

Soak collard greens in a large sink or steel bowl. Pick through the greens and discard yellow leaves and any thick stems. Dry and cut out the thicker stem of the collard greens. Stack 3-4 leaves and roll the leaves crosswise into tiny strips or chop into 1/4" strips.

In a large pot over medium heat, heat the oil. Sauté the onions until slightly softened, about 4-5 minutes, then add the red pepper flakes, and garlic, cook another minute. Add collard greens and cook another minute. Add the vegetable stock, coconut liquid aminos and balsamic vinegar, cover and bring to a simmer. Add filtered water as needed. Cook until greens are tender, about 40 minutes. Add or garnish with tomatoes and season with salt and freshly ground black pepper.

RECIPE 411:

Did you know food historians date collard greens back to prehistoric times? Collard greens are members of the cabbage family. These greens are immune boosting and full of iron, Vitamin A, Vitamin C and other hearty nutrients. Although many people associate greens with southern African-American culture, the reality is different. Here's the deal. Collard greens are popular plants with a rich soulful history. The Romans and Portuguese have long used collard greens. Even so, I know you might want to hear more about the southern variety of greens that has hammocks or smoked turkey meat added to the collard greens, or the cornbread for dunking but you'll be shocked to know how "detoxelicious" this dish is without any added meat. It's just the African slaves and Native Americans shared ideas on how to make the collard greens more flavorful in the South. So, from my grandma table to yours, eat "detoxeliciousl," without any complex animal meat proteins.

TIP: It takes a lot of will power and patient to get rid of the grit that loves to cling to these green leaves. Because rinsing is not enough, I recommend you soak them ahead of time. You can fill a clean sink with cold water and sprinkle the greens with salt. I recommend you clean the sink again then let the greens soak one to two more times. After soaking, then remove the coarse stem from the leaves with a knife. Cleaning greens can be fun for the kids since they have little fingers. It helps them to understand the concept of "farm-to-table" foods.

Detoxelicious Day 7

EVERY DAY IS A NEW BEGINNING

Today is a good day to press the reset button. Let's start the day with gratitude from the moment we open our eyes and think about getting out of bed and brushing our teeth. With every sunrise, there is a sunset. With every inhale, there is an exhale in life. With every attachment to a person, money or a possession, there will be detachment. Even in yoga, we hold on to a pose and we let go. Recognize the dichotomy of life experiences. See the beauty with the illumination of awareness in all things. So be patient with yourself and make a fresh new start or beginning.

"When you inhale, you are taking strength from God. When you exhale, it represents the service you are giving to the world." - Geeta Iyengar

Daily Detox Pose 7: Shoulder Stand

Key Actions: Lie down on a folded blanket. Place your shoulder blades along the lower edge width distance apart. Lay your arms on the floor alongside your torso, then bend your knees and set your feet against the floor with the heels close to your sit bones. Press your arms into mat, push your feet away from the floor towards the ceiling. Continue to lift legs until your pelvis is over the shoulders. Walk the hands up your back while keeping the elbows grounded to the mat. Hold for 30 seconds. Gradually, add 5 to 10 seconds every day until you can hold for 3 minutes. Sanskrit name: Salamba Sarvangasana

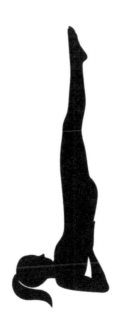

Benefits: This extended pose calms the nervous systems and helps to relieve stress and mild depression. It also stimulates the thyroid and abdominal organs. It also improves digestion and offers relief to some asthma and sinusitis sufferers.

BREAKFAST

Citrus Apple Carrot Smoothie

Serves 1 to 2 people

INGREDIENTS

- 2 large carrots
- 1 apple, cored and chopped
- ½ cup frozen pineapple
- Juice of ½ lemon
- Pinch each ground cinnamon and ground ginger

INSTRUCTIONS

Total time: 4 to 7 minutes Place all ingredients inside a high-speed blender. Add filtered water until water is slightly above the same eye level of the solid, chopped apple and carrots. Blend until smooth. Pour into glass and enjoy.

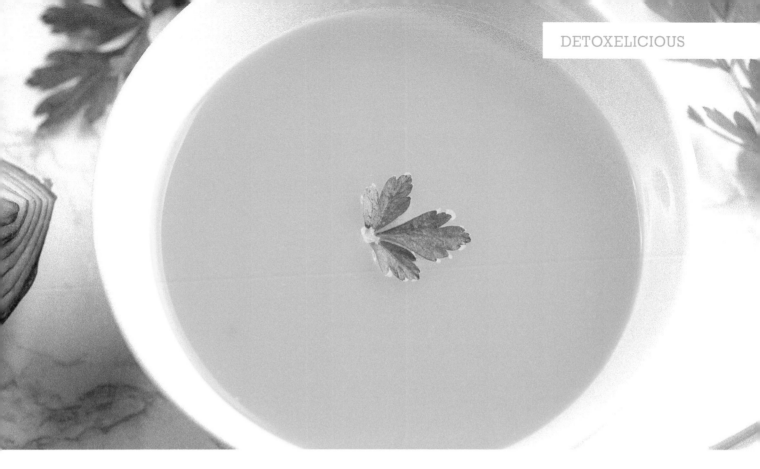

LUNCH

Vegan Butternut Squash Soup

Serves 4 to 6 people

INGREDIENTS

- 2 tablespoons olive oil
- 2 large garlic cloves
- 1 cup yellow onion, finely chopped
- 2 celery stalks, chopped
- 2 large carrots, finely chopped

- 8 cups chopped butternut squash (peeled, seeded and chopped into cubes)
- 4 cups vegetable stock
- 1 tablespoon coconut liquid amino
- 1 cup plain unsweetened cashew milk
- Salt to taste
- Pepper to taste

INSTRUCTIONS

In a large pot over medium heat, add the olive oil and saute the garlic, onions and celery, stirring often until soft and translucent, about 5 minutes.

Add carrots, butter squash, vegetable stock and coconut liquid amino. Bring to a boil, then reduce the heat to low and simmer until all the vegetables are tender, about 35 to 40 minutes. Transfer vegetable mixture in batches to a blender and process until smooth. Return new smooth mixture back to the large pot. Stir in the cashew milk, salt and pepper and cook until desired consistency. Continue to add more cashew milk as desired. Serve hot. Garnish with a basil leaf and/or olive oil.

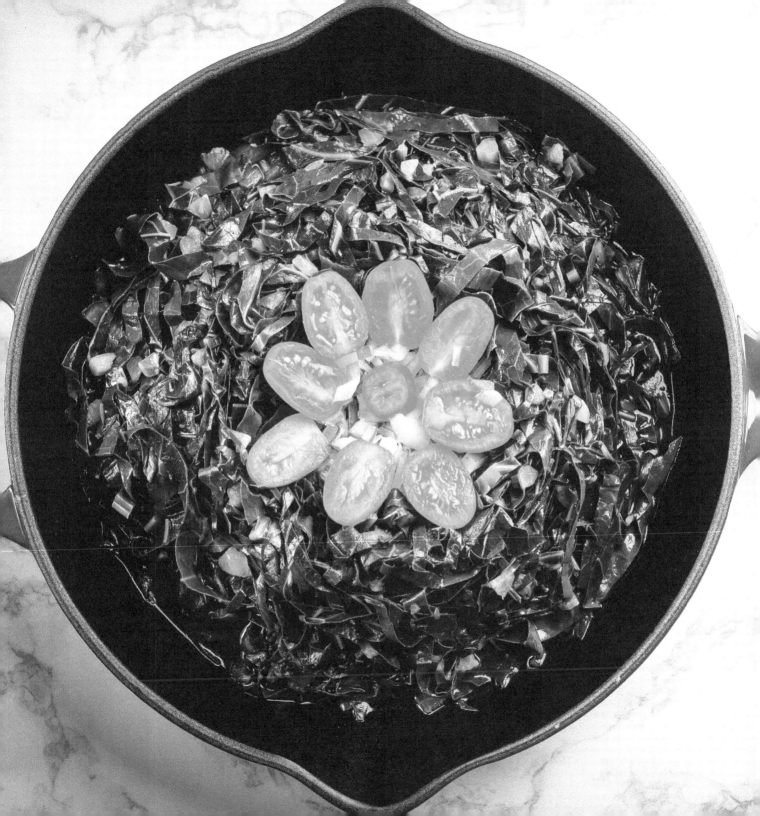

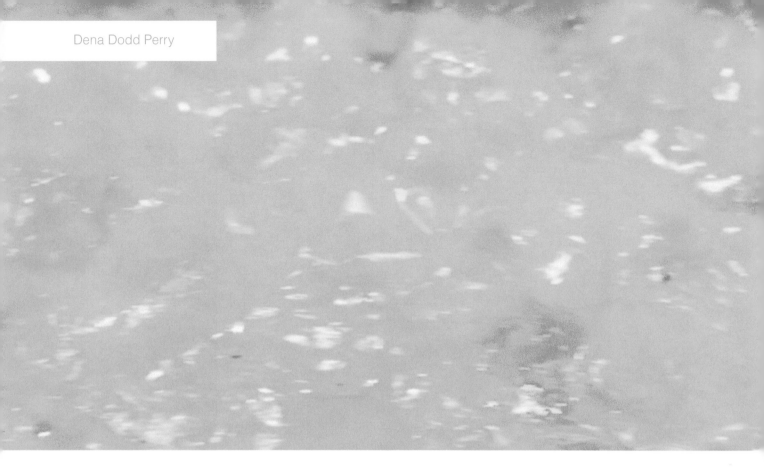

Dena Dodd Perry

DINNER

Vegan Mac & Cheese

INGREDIENTS

- 1 cup raw cashews
- one pound bean-based elbow pasta (or substitute whole wheat elbows)
- 1 ½ tablespoons avocado oil or vegan butter
- 1 large shallot or 1 small onion, peeled
- 3 tablespoons fresh lemon juice
- 3 cloves garlic, degermed
- ½ teaspoon each onion powder, dry mustard powder, and fine sea salt

- ¼ teaspoon ground turmeric
- 3 tablespoons nutritional yeast flakes
- 1 pinch red pepper flakes

INSTRUCTIONS

In small bowl, soak the cashews in 2 cups of water for two hours. Drain and set aside.

Prepare pasta according to package directions. While pasta is cooking, prepare sauce.

In a high-speed blender or food processor, combine cashews with ¾ cup warm water, shallot or onion, lemon juice, garlic, spices, nutritional yeast and red pepper flakes. Purée until mixture is completely smooth, scraping down sides as needed. If needed, thin with a tablespoon or two of water.

When pasta is tender, drain and rinse it, then return to pasta pot and stir in the cheese sauce. Season to taste with salt and pepper. Serve warm.

RECIPE 411:

Many grocers now carry boxed and frozen varieties of vegan mac & cheese. However, you are adding unnecessary carbohydrates to your detox diet should you use the store-bought variety for your cleanse. This recipe has the added powerful antioxidants from garlic, lemon juice and turmeric. So enjoy a healthier mac & cheese for this week. Stay strong!

Detoxelicious Day 8

PEACE BEGINS WHEN EXPECTATIONS END.

Everyone has a public life and a private inner life. The public life is what we share with others, how we show up at work or move about around strangers. The inner life is made up of our feelings, thoughts, images and motives. Only you and God know what's going on inside of you. Many times, we set expectations of how things are supposed to be without accepting how they really are. Once we release expectations and observe, we begin to see situations more clearly. We make better choices for ourselves. Like many women, I made a bad choice with a particular boyfriend. I admit that he was a bad choice in my life. I had expectations of how a guy should treat me and he did not meet those expectations. I thought I needed him in my life to experience true happiness, but I came to realize I did not. Once I realized that we were not aligned energetically and let go of my expectations, my life began to fall into place.

Are you at peace with yourself? God is looking at the inner life. You can't fake the funk with God. And, you know what? If a certain choice costs you your peace, then it's not worth your energy. It's too expensive. Be selective with what and who you give your energy to. Don't give energy to ignorant people or what they think of you. Ask God to give you peace with your choices and every aspect of your life. In other words, I made peace my choices and reminded myself that my best is good enough. (A glass of wine is optional and may help us cope as well!) Peace begins when your expectations end. Give yourself a break. Restore balance. No one taught us how to outgrow toxic relationships. Detox from unhealthy food and people so new, healthier choices can fill its space.

Daily Detox Pose 8: Plow Pose

Key Actions: Enter Shoulder Stand first. From shoulder stand exhale and bend from the hip joints to the slowly pull your toes up and over until your toes meet or are near the mat. Lift the top of your thighs and your tailbone toward the ceiling. Draw your chin away from your sternum or chest. Hold for 1 to 3 minutes then roll down onto your back, or roll out of the pose entirely. Use several blankets to ease any tension on the neck. If you still feel tension take your legs up the wall for inverted lake. Sanskrit Name: Halasana

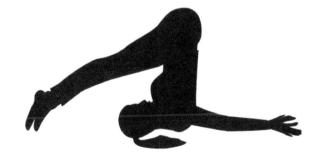

Benefits: This plow pose is capable of draining the accumulated lymph fluid from the legs and re-circulating it through the body. This benefits the immune system. Inverting is also good for increasing metabolism and stimulating the thyroid gland.

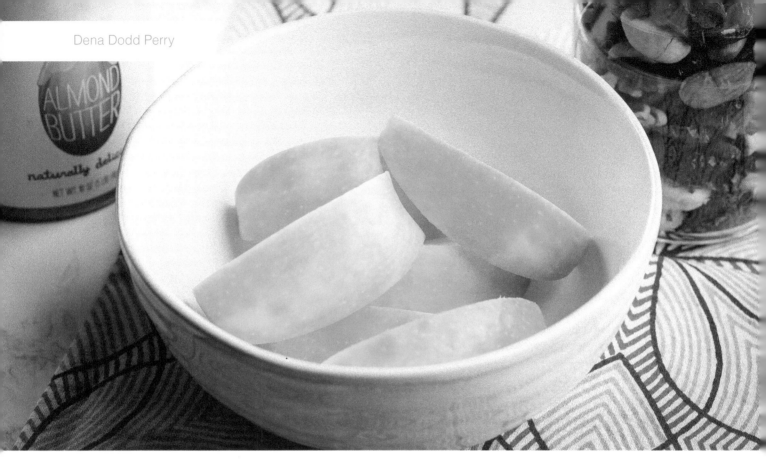

BREAKFAST

Apple Kale Smoothie

Serves 1 to 2 people.

INGREDIENTS

- 1 cup of unsweetened vanilla almond milk
- 1 cup chopped kale, rinsed thoroughly
- ½ cup carrot chunks
- ½ peeled avocado

- ½ cup chopped frozen mangoes
- 1 tablespoon chia seeds
- Filtered water

INSTRUCTIONS

Total time: 4 to 7 minutes

Place all ingredients inside a high-speed blender. Add filtered water if needed to thin. Blend all ingredients for about 1 minutes until smooth. Pour into glass and enjoy.

RECIPE 411

I know you might be mad at me for adding kale in this one. I don't know why people say hurtful things like, "Want to go for a run? Or, try this kale?" Hilarious! But, kale is truly packed with much-needed fiber for your body. It will keep you full and regular. Just always add a scoop of avocado to cut out the grittiness from the kale. It's life-changing, for real!

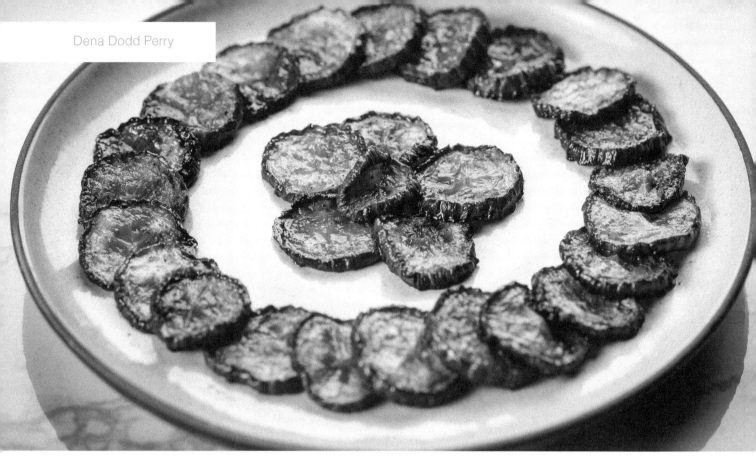

Dena Dodd Perry

LUNCH

Oven-Fried Okra

Serves 1 to 2 people

INGREDIENTS

- 1-pound fresh okra stem ends trimmed, sliced into ½ inch thick rounds
- 2 tablespoon olive oil
- ½ teaspoon hot pepper sauce
- 1 cup garbanzo flour
- 1 teaspoon lemon pepper
- ½ teaspoon garlic salt water as needed

INSTRUCTIONS

1. Fill a large steel pot ¾ full with salted waterl. Boil okra until tender for about 4 minutes, drain well.

2. Mix 1 tablespoon olive oil, 1 tablespoon water and hot pepper sauce; add okra to the bowl.

3. Preheat oven to 425F degrees. In a large bag or Ziploc, mix the remaining olive oil with the garbanzo flour. Add 1 tablespoon water, salt and pepper to the bag until the consistency is like thick soup. Using a wire spatula, gather the okra from flour mixture and allow excess mixture to drip back into bowl. Add okra to flour mixture in bag. Gently turn bag to coat okra evenly.

4. On a nonstick baking sheet or large shallow pan, spread the okra in a single layer. Bake until golden brown, about 10-14 minutes. Makes 6 side dish servings or 3 mono meals.

RECIPE 411:

Okra probably originated near Ethiopia, and was cultivated by the ancient Egyptians by the 12th century B.C. Its cultivation spread throughout North Africa and the Middle East. The seed pods were eaten cooked, and the seeds were toasted and ground, used as a coffee substitute (and still is).

Okra came to the Caribbean and the U.S. in the 1700s, probably brought by slaves from West Africa, and was introduced to Western Europe soon after. In Louisiana, the Creoles learned from slaves the use of okra (gumbo) to thicken soups, and it is now an essential ingredient in Creole Gumbo. It grows well in the southern United States where there is little frost.

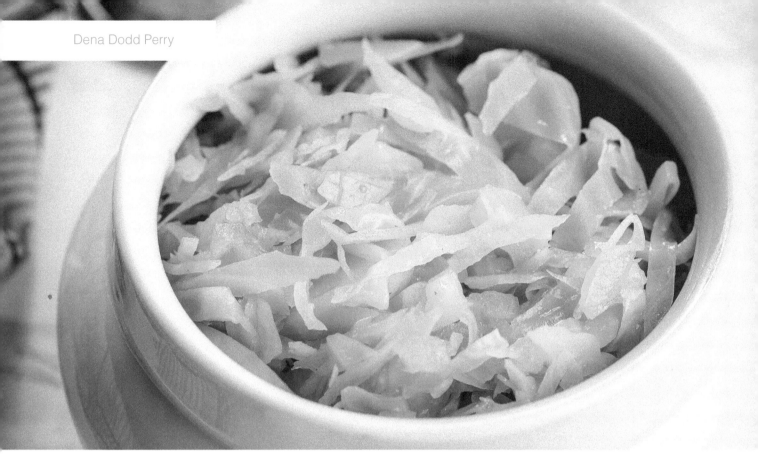

DINNER

Cabbage & Vegan Bacon Soup

INGREDIENTS

- 1 tablespoon olive oil
- One package field roast vegan bacon
- 1 medium yellow onion, chopped
- 1 stalk celery, sliced thin,
- 1-quart organic vegetable broth
- 1 Bay leaf

96

- 2 large carrots, diced
- 1-pound green cabbage, coarsely shredded
- 1 tablespoon fresh lemon juice
- 2 tablespoon coconut liquid aminos
- ½ teaspoon lemon pepper
- ½ teaspoon cayenne pepper
- 1 teaspoon caraway seed
- 2 tablespoons parsley, chopped

INSTRUCTIONS

In a large pan, fry the vegan bacon in 1 tablespoon of olive oil or coconut oil. Once slightly browned on both sides, remove from pan and place onto paper towel to drain any excess oil. Next, cook onion and celery just until onion is transparent. Add broth, bacon and bay leaf; bring to a simmer. Cook several minutes to season broth.

Stir in carrots, cabbage and lemon juice, coconut aminos, lemon pepper, cayenne pepperand caraway seeds into broth mixture. Simmer all vegetables until tender which may take 10-15 minutes. Remove and throw away bay leaf.

Cut vegan bacon into small bit size pieces, return meat to soup pot. Add caraway seeds and mix well. Cook just until heated for about another 10-15 minutes. Use a ladle to serve in ceramic bowls. Sprinkle with parsley and serve.

RECIPE 411:

I love this little variation on cabbage with the detoxifying benefits of cayenne pepper. As you may know, the first detox drinks were lemon water with cayenne pepper mixed in. This recipe takes that historical concept to a whole new soul-food level.

Detoxelicious Day 9

BE A WARRIOR FOR LOVE AND PEACE

Life is difficult so we must fight the good fight. We live in a crazy world. In most countries, violence and poverty rates are escalating year by year in most countries. If we are appalled by violence, unfairness, injustice or bigotry of any kind, we must speak truth to power. It's important to build compassion and trust before speaking your truth even to the most disparaging characters. Disarm. Organize your thoughts. We must have the courage to speak even it makes your voice shake a little. A little nervousness is good for the soul. If your message is persistently filled with hope, love and peace, it should be well-received by the universe. Love is always on the good side of righteousness in this world we live in. We become conspirators to hate when we become silent to things that matter in humanity. So, create balance from the good things happening in your environment and create solutions to the things you can change in your environment. Diffuse the power of the problem by discussing your problem. Be a problem solver. Speak truth to power for the sake of love and peace towards solutions.

How do we achieve love and peace? Those moments are achieved when there is no holding back your emotions because you have the lightness of a clear mind. When this clear mind occurs, we know our decisions and choices are paying off real dividends. Those dividends show up as clear acceptance. Peace comes to us often as healing after knowing that wisdom comes to us from having clearer knowledge. We do this from a place of love, not of fear. Fear rears its ugly head as racism, jealousy, envy, and vindictiveness. Due to karmic forces, more fear begets bad behavior. Conversely, more love begets good behavior. Action derived from love is brave and creative. Fear does not produce the power to create, alternatively it craves destruction. May we all understand that love is the prerequisite to healing. When we heal from our thoughts and choices, we achieve peace. As an added bonus, a calm mind through meditation paves the way to your true power. So, there is true loving power in silence. The power of the universe has your back with peace and loves a calm believer of prayer and meditation. Be a warrior for love and peace.

Assignment: Pick any sentence in any foreword here or elsewhere from a book you love and repeat the sentence to yourself for 1-2 minutes. Breathe in your nose and exhale through your mouth. Enjoy your meditation.

Daily Detox Pose 9: Boat Pose

Key Actions: Sit on the floor with your legs fully extended forward. Press your hands onto the floor next to you. Lift through the top of the sternum and lean your torso back slightly. Lift the chest towards the ceiling or sky. Do not round the back. Exhale and bend your knees, then lift your feet off the floor. Lengthen your tailbone into the mat and crown of the head back along a 45degree angle. If possible, you can slowly straighten your knees, raising the tips of your toes slightly above the level of eyes. For a modified version, keep your knees bent and hold to your lower thighs while lifting the shins parallel to the floor.

Go slowly and do 15 reps depending upon your strength. On the last boat pose, hold for 30-60 seconds. Sanskrit name: Navasana

Benefit: The benefits are that boat pose works to clear the liver, gall bladder and spleen. These will tone your abs and get you back into shape quickly. This will nicely build your core abdominal muscles when done on a regular basis.

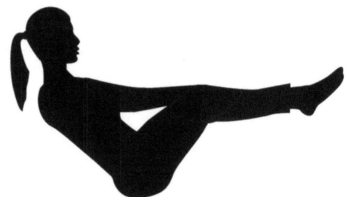

BREAKFAST

Tango Mango Smoothie

Serves 1 to 2 people.

INGREDIENTS

- 1 cup chopped frozen mango
- ½ cup almond or coconut milk
- ½ cup of pineapple
- ½ avocado, peeled and scooped Filtered water

INSTRUCTIONS

Total time: 4 to 7 minutes

Place all ingredients inside a high-speed blender. Add filtered water until liquid level is slightly above frozen solid level measurement in the blender. Blend all ingredients for about 1 minute until smooth. Pour into glass and enjoy.

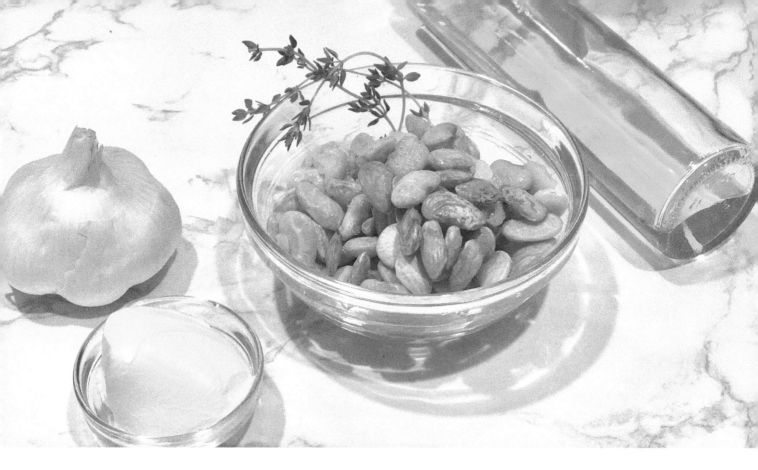

LUNCH

Mo' Butter Bean Soup

Serves 4 to 6 people

INGREDIENTS

- 1-pound dried butter beans
- 1 cup chopped vegan bacon
- 1 package mixed vegetables
- 3 medium scallions, chopped

- 2 teaspoons dried thyme
- 6 cups organic vegetable broth
- Filtered water
- Garnish with chopped tomatoes

INSTRUCTIONS

Rinse the butter beans in a colander. Discard any beans that look damaged. In a large steel bowl, soak the bean overnight in filtered water.

Drain the beans.

In a large soup pot, fry the vegan bacon until crispy. Remove bacon and break into small bite size pieces. Combine all ingredients including the butter beans, vegan bacon bits, mixed vegetable, scallions, thyme, broth and desired cups of water. Simmer on low to medium heat for 2 hours. For a creamy less bulky texture, simply puree half the beans in a high-speed blender and return the puree back to the pot. Or, use a potato masher to mash up half the beans. In either case, serve hot and garnish with chopped tomatoes.

This is a naturally creamy soup which is rich and detoxelicious. Butter beans are in the lima bean family. It's rich with fiber, calcium and other great nutrients. Enjoy this rather filling option on your detoxelicious journey.

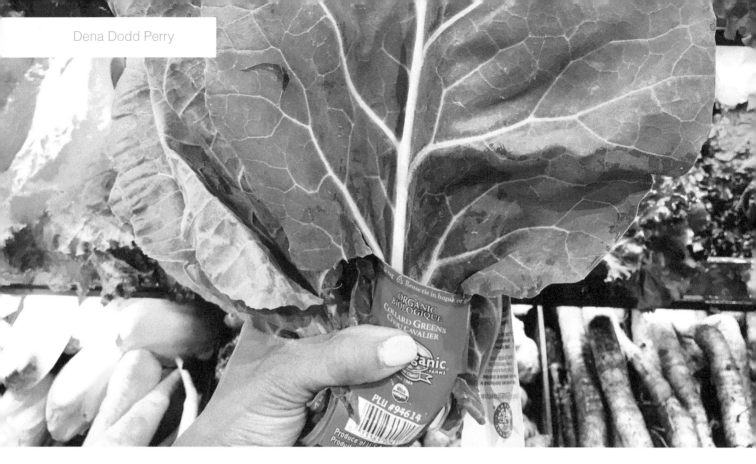

DINNER

Avocado Collards Wraps

INGREDIENTS

- 2 ripe avocados, skin and pit removed
- ½ cup chopped tomatoes, no seeds or extra juice
- Juice of one lime
- ½ medium onion, chopped
- 2 tablespoons olive oil
- 2 teaspoon garlic, minced

- Salt to taste
- 8 large collard green leaves
- Few sprigs of cilantro or parsley

INSTRUCTIONS

In medium bowl, mash avocados in a bowl. Mash avocados, tomatoes, lime juice, onions and garlic until the texture is chunky smooth. (Alternatively, use a food processor if you prefer silky smooth texture.) Once your guacamole is completely mashed, cover and set aside in the refrigerator.

Remove the freshest looking collard leaves from the bunch. Trim off any the white stalk and any damaged portion of the leaf. Soak leaves in warm water and 2 tablespoons of vinegar for 5 minutes or more. Dry each leaf. Take a dollop of guacamole, drizzle with olive oil, and place lengthwise along the center of the collard leaf. Roll lengthwise then cut crosswise. You can eat the wraps as boats or cut crosswise into smaller pin wheels or mini-boats. Either way, it's some quick green goodness. Just add more seasonings or cilantro to taste.

RECIPE 411:

You can buy freshly made guacamole from most health food stores. It just tastes even better if you make this at home.

Detoxelicious Day 10

TRUST YOUR JOURNEY
My yoga teacher guru, trained by BKS Iyengar, once told me to practice 1000 times and ask one question rather than ask 1000 questions and practice once.

I've developed such a fond appreciation of life experiences such as yoga, math, dancing, writing, debate and so many other talents. After training under this yoga style for a year, I'm now so appreciative of the journey. I've learned to enjoy the process without expectations of any desired outcome. If you do this in every aspect of work or personal life, somehow the experience becomes so much more enjoyable. In summary, you finished the detox cleanse. Maybe it's not so much about the destination, then it is about your journey. We must learn to embrace struggle for it will likely be our greatest teacher. Practice non-judgment in challenging situations because we don't know what challenges people are facing. Gather your strength and trust your journey. It's all there to teach us something new about ourselves. Give daily gratitude and trust your journey. Congratulations!

Daily Detox Pose 10: Bridge Pose

Key Actions: Lie down with your back on the floor. Place a blanket parallel to your shoulders to protect your neck. Bend your knees and set your feet on the floor with your heels comfortably placed parallel to the mat. Slowly, lift the buttocks off the floor while pressing your inner feet and arms firmly into the floor. Hold and lengthen the tailbone towards the knees. Lift the chin slightly up away from the chest. Broaden the collar bone muscles. Hold for 30 seconds to 1 minute. Slow release one vertebrae at a time. Sanskrit name: Setu Bandha Sarvangasana

Benefits: Open the chest to counteract occurrences with congestion and stagnation. Back bends are also very useful to increase metabolism.

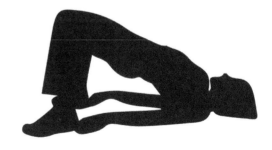

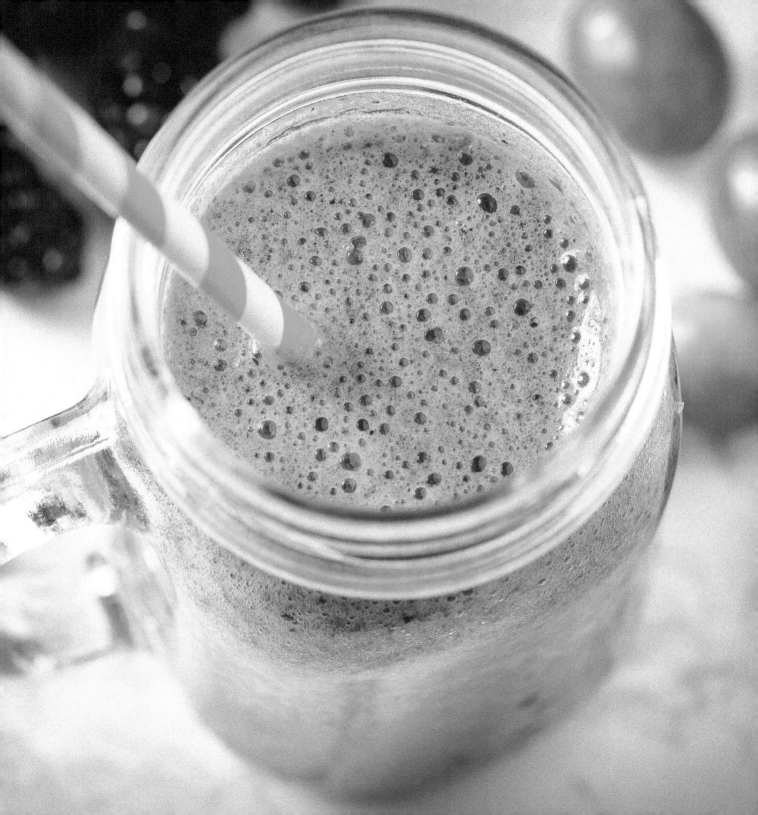

BREAKFAST

Berry Merry Smoothie

Serves 1 to 2 people

INGREDIENTS

- 1 cup frozen mixed organic berries
- 1 cup organic spinach
- ½ cup strawberries
- 1 tablespoon grounded flaxseeds
- 1 cup organic orange juice

INSTRUCTIONS

Place all ingredients into high speed blender. Blend until smooth. If too thick, remember to add more filtered water. Pour into a large glass and enjoy.

RECIPE 411:

Did you know dark fruits and vegetables can make your urine and poop dark? Well, sorry to get so personal but it's true. Your excretions can become the same color as the food you eat. So, don't be alarmed like Oprah was. She called her doctor when she looked in the toilet after eating so many beets. Yikes! Just calm down and enjoy the added benefits of feeling healthy and more energetic.

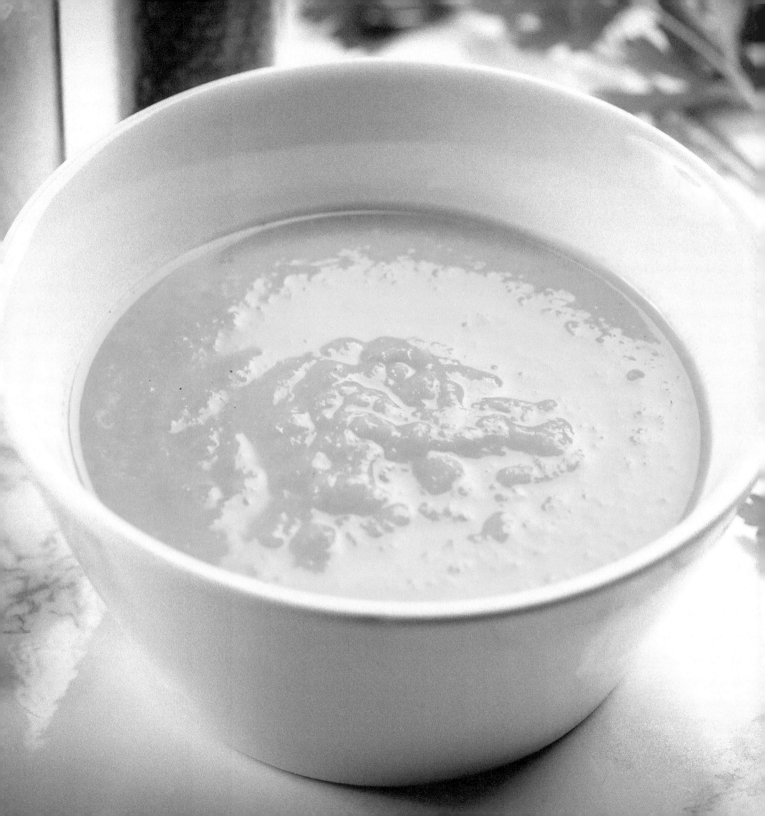

LUNCH

Ginger Carrot Soup

Serves 4 people

INGREDIENTS

- ¼ cup vegan butter
- 1 whole yellow onion, chopped
- 1 tablespoon fresh ginger, finely chopped
- 2 teaspoons minced garlic
- 1-pound organic carrots, peeled and chopped
- 2 tomatoes, seeded, chopped
- 1 teaspoon grated lemon peel, grated
- 3 cups vegetable stock or broth
- 1 tablespoons fresh lemon juice
- Salt and pepper to taste
- 1 small carrot, peeled, grated

INSTRUCTIONS

Place butter in heavy soup pot over medium heat. Add onion, sauté 4 minutes. Add ginger and garlic and cook for 3 minutes. Add chopped carrots, tomatoes, and lemon peel. Cook for an additional minute. Add 3 cups stock and bring to boil. Reduce heat, cover partially and simmer until carrots are very tender, about 20 minutes. Cool slightly.

Puree soup in batches in a high-speed blender. Return soup to pot. Mix in lemon juice. Season with salt and pepper. Bring soup to a gentle boil. Thin the soup with more stock if needed. Serve with a ladle into soup bowls and garnish with grated carrot.

RECIPE 411:

This is a must-have during your detox week. The natural combination of the carrot's sweetness with the spiciness of the ginger is a match made in heaven. You can make this one ahead of time and just reheat when needed. Use a steel pot if storing in the refrigerator. Enjoy your carrot-ginger soup that is rich with vitamin A from beta carotene, biotin and anti-inflammatory benefits.

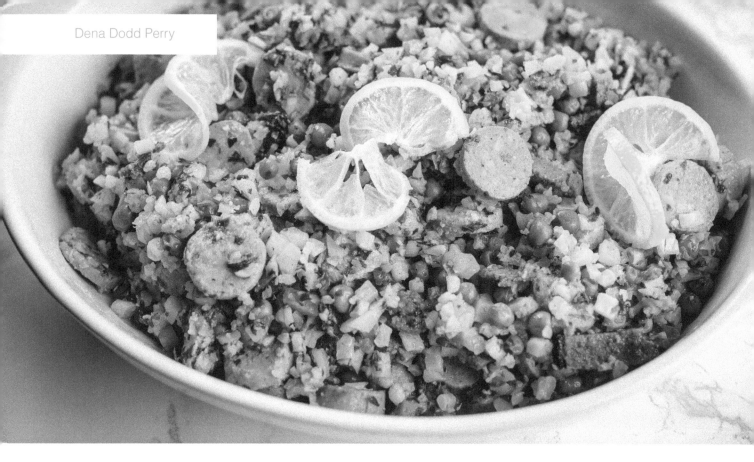

DINNER

Vegan Cauli-Jambalaya Skillet
Serves 4 to 6

INGREDIENTS

- (2-pound) head cauliflower, trimmed and cut into small florets (7 to 8 cups)
- 2 to 4 tablespoons extra-virgin olive oil
- 1 pound vegan Spanish chorizo
- 1½ teaspoon kosher salt
- 1 small yellow onion, diced

- garlic cloves, finely chopped
- 14.5-ounce can whole tomatoes, with juice, crushed by hand
- 2 cups vegetable stock
- ½ tsp. saffron threads (It comes in a little bottle.)
- 1 cup frozen peas, thawed
- ¼ cup finely chopped flat-leaf parsley'
- 1 tablespoon coconut liquid aminos
- 1 lemon, cut into wedges

INSTRUCTIONS

Using a food processor fitted with a metal blade, pulse cauliflower in batches until reduced to the size of large grains; you should have about 4 packed cups. Or, better yet, see if your local health food store sells them in the pre-packed cauliflower rice packets. Get it. Set aside.

In a large, deep skillet, heat 2 tablespoons oil over medium-high heat. Add vegan chorizo and cook until sizzling and golden, 2 to 3 minutes. Using a slotted spoon, transfer chorizo to a large plate; set aside.

Return skillet to medium-high heat. Add cauliflower and salt and cook, stirring occasionally, until golden, about 5 minutes. Add onion and cook, scraping up any browned bits, until soft and translucent, about 5 minutes. Stir in garlic and cook 1 minute more. Stir in tomatoes, stock, and saffron and bring just to a boil.

Scatter chorizo over top of skillet contents. Reduce heat to medium, cover, and cook until thickened and fragrant about 5 minutes.

Stir in peas, and parsley and coconut aminos. Serve immediately, with lemon wedges on the side. You'll love me for this recipe too!

AFTERWORD

Why did I write this book? My mother died from a cardiovascular angiogram medical mishap. I wanted to share ideas on making incremental lifestyle changes that lead to better health outcomes. First, I've interviewed many doctors within the last two years. Some have taken this detox cleanse. I especially love convincing family friends who are doctors to take the detox cleanse. Second, I received my degree in Industrial Engineering and Management Sciences in 1990. This degree involved specialized training in probability and statistics and market research. For example, in 2000, my economic retail trade study of a large suburban town in Illinois revealed the fact that food deserts existed within the southern region, meaning residents had to travel a long distance before reaching a grocery store. The work resulted in having the town land their first-ever Panera Bread. Pursuing better wellness outcomes is nothing new for me. In closing, I know a healthier lifestyle might not be easy for some of us but just know, it's worth it to make the change even if it's just for 10-days. One doctor told me that "it is a really good idea to give your liver and kidneys a break." Detoxifying with fiber-rich, delicious plant-based foods should be a lifestyle. It makes good sense. Recognize. Reset. Realize your results from the detox process as shown on Page 32. You matter. You got this.

REFERENCES

"African Mango (Irvingia Gabonensis) Benefits & Information." Herbwisdom. Herbwisdom, 03 Feb. 2015. Web. 01 May 2016.

Begley, Sharon. "Why Chemicals Called Obesogens May Make You Fat." Newsweek. Newsweek, 10 Sept. 2009. Web. 03 May 2016.

Cohen, Suzy. "Calcium D-glucarate: A Novel Way to Eliminate Toxins." Total Health Magazine. The Well- ness Imperative People. Web. 30 April. 2016.

"Dirty Dozen Endocrine Disruptors." EWG. Environmental Working Group, 28 Oct. 2013. Web. 01 May 2016.

"Exposure to Endocrine Disruptors during Pregnancy Affects the Brain Two Generations Later, Rat Study Shows." ScienceDaily. Endocrine Society, 05 Mar. 2015. Web. 03 May 2016.

Grens, Kerry. "Obesogens." The Scientist. The Scientist, 01 Nov. 2015. Web. "Health Benefits of Taking Probiotics - Harvard Health." Harvard Health. 01 Sept. 2005. Web. 01 May 2016.

Holtcamp, Wendee. "Obesogens: An Environmental Link to Obesity." Environmental Health Perspectives. National Institute of Environmental Health Sciences, Feb. 2012. Web. 10 Apr. 2016.

"How Does Fiber Affect Blood Glucose Levels?" Joslin Diabetes Center. Harvard Medical School. Web. 30 Apr. 2016.

Mason, Russ. "Environmental Toxins and Weight Gain: The Link. An Interview with Paula Baillie-Hamilton MB, BS, Dphil." Positive Health Online. Positive Health Online, Feb. 2006. Web. 30 Apr. 2016.

McPartland. Iennifer "Do These Chemicals Make Me Look Fat7" EDF Health. Environmental Defense Fund. 19 Jan. 2011. Web. 01 May 2016.

Mercer. Sarah Jane. "The Three-Day Detox Plan Anyone Can Do." VegNews RSS. Veg News. 16 Mar. 2016. Web. 01 May 2016.

Meyer. Amy, MD. "The Auto Immune Solution – Prevent and Reversing The Full Spectrum of Inflammatory Symptoms & Diseases." Harper One. 2017

Ng. Marie. "Global. Regional. and National Prevalence of Overweight and Obesity in Children and Adults during 1980-2013: A Systematic Analysis for the Global Burden of Disease Study 2013." Thelancet. Elsevier. 28 May 2014. Web. 15 Apr. 2016.

"Overweight and Obesity Statistics." Weight-control Information Network (2012). National Institutes of Health. Oct. 2012. Web.

Perrine. Stephen. and Heather Hurlock. "Fat Epidemic Linked to Chemicals Run Amok." Msnbc.com. Men's Health. 08 Mar. 2010. Web. 01 May 2016.

Seshadri.Sudha. Article et al. "The Lifetime Risk of Stroke." 37:345-50. 2006.

Smith. Michael W. MD. "Probiotics and Prebiotics: Ask the Nutritionist on WebMD." WebMD. WebMD. Web. 18 Apr. 2016.

Woodruff. Teresa. PhD. United States Public Health Statistics Presentation. The Women's Health Research Institute. 2017.

"The Vast Majority of American Adults Are Overweight or Obese. and Weight Is a Growing

Problem among US Children." Healthdata. Institute for Health Metrics and Evaluation Web 01 May 2016

SUPPLEMENTS

http://www.nature.com/nature/journal/v473/n7346/abs/nature09944.html

http://articles.mercola.com/sites/articles/archive/2012/06/27/probiotics-gut-health-impact.aspx http://www.scientificamerican.com/article/how-gut-bacteria-help-make-us-fat-and-thin/ http://www.medicalnewstoday.com/releases/250221.php https://draxe.com/prebiotics/ http://drlwilson.com/ARTICLES/FLORA.htm http://www.webmd.com/digestive-disorders/news/20140820/your-gut-bacteria#1 http://www.mindbodygreen.com/0-10908/9-signs-you-have-a-leaky-gut.html

http://www.drdavidwilliams.com/gut-health-and-the-benefits-of-traditional-fermented-foods/ http://health.usnews.com/health-news/blogs/eat-run/2014/03/06/leaky-gut-what-it-is-and-howto-heal-it http://www.jillcarnahan.com/2014/07/07/leaky-gut-syndrome-linked-manyautoimmune-diseases/